D0861542

By H. IRVING HANCOCK

———

Jiu-Jitsu Combat Tricks

Life at West Point

Physical Training for Business Men

Complete Kano Jiu-Jitsu

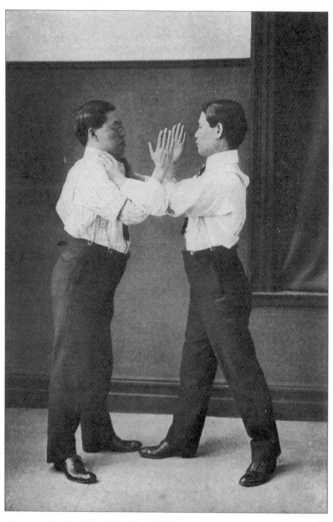

Nº 1. ONE OF THE SIMPLEST FORMS OF THROW-OFF OF THROAT-HOLD.

Jiu-Jitsu
Combat Tricks

A Classic Guide to
the Ancient Art

By

H. Irving Hancock

Author of "Physical Training for Women by Japanese Methods,"
"Physical Culture Life," "Life at West Point," etc.

Illustrated with Thirty-two Photographs
Taken from Life by A. B. Phelan and Others

SPORTS
PUBLISHING

Sports Publishing books may be purchased in bulk at special discounts for sales promotion, corporate gifts, fund-raising, or educational purposes. Special editions can also be created to specifications. For details, contact the Special Sales Department, Sports Publishing, 307 West 36th Street, 11th Floor, New York, NY 10018 or sportspubbooks@skyhorsepublishing.com.

Sports Publishing® is a registered trademark of Skyhorse Publishing, Inc.®, a Delaware corporation.

Visit our website at www.sportspubbooks.com.

10 9 8 7 6 5 4 3 2 1

Library of Congress Cataloging-in-Publication Data is on file.

ISBN: 978-1-61321-210-3

Printed in China

INTRODUCTION

IT is but a few years ago that *jiu-jitsu* was unknown to the Western world. To-day the name is understood very generally, in English-speaking countries, to refer to that mysterious art of self-defence by which the Japanese prove antagonists whom it is impossible to defeat in physical encounter. To some extent, too, a little knowledge of this strange art has come to us. Within the next few years it is to be expected that *jiu-jitsu* will be as well understood by us as boxing is to-day.

A knowledge of the Japanese art reduces boxing from a science of defence to the status of an excellent exercise. The well-trained *jiu-jitsian* is able to meet and to defeat the fistic expert at all points. In this volume much attention has been paid to the methods by which the Japanese overcomes the exponent of ring work.

In scope the feats described in this volume

comprise all that is essential in *jiu-jitsu* for purposes of personal encounter. Much that would be of interest only under Japanese conditions of life has been omitted. The tricks selected for analysis in this volume are those that are of the most value to the man of Anglo-Saxon heritage in matters of fighting.

Without doubt it will be urged that some of the Japanese feats explained in the following pages are, in the language of the ring, "foul." But fighting is an ugly business from the nature of things, and the Japanese contend that any means that brings victory is justifiable. It may be added that few men defeated by a *jiu-jitsian* are disabled for a period longer than a few moments following defeat. The lacerations and contusions that follow fisticuffs are unknown in Japan, where to disfigure an opponent would be considered a disgrace to the victor. *Jiu-jitsu*, while stern work, is the essence of politeness; it is aimed to show a bully the folly of fighting.

The greatest charm of all about *jiu-jitsu* is that it does not call for the employment of great strength. The weaker man, if skilled, is

Introduction

able to vanquish his stronger but unversed opponent.   The art has a history of more than twenty-five centuries, and, during its long course of evolution, *jiu-jitsu* has been perfected as the art of the smaller, weaker man.

Daily practice in this novel physical work makes rapidly for agility of body and of mind, and for great physical endurance.   The Japanese soldier, sailor, and policeman take a compulsory government course in *jiu-jitsu*.   The physical performances of the Japanese in their war with Russia should be sufficient to establish even seemingly extravagant claims for the value of *jiu-jitsu* as the best system of bodily training known to the world.

H. IRVING HANCOCK.

NEW YORK, July 25, 1904.

CONTENTS

CHAPTER I.

CHAPTER II.

CHAPTER III.

CHAPTER IV.

CHAPTER V.

Contents

Contents

Contents

CHAPTER XVI.

ILLUSTRATIONS

Illustrations

JIU-JITSU COMBAT TRICKS

CHAPTER I

PRELIMINARY TRAINING—HOW TO
STRENGTHEN THE HANDS FOR ATTACK,
AND HOW TO TOUGHEN THE VULNERABLE
PARTS FOR DEFENCE — PRACTICE MUST
BE CONSTANT UNTIL PERFORMANCE OF
THE TRICKS BECOMES SECOND NATURE—
DON'T BE IN A HURRY TO "SHOW OFF"
A NEW TRICK TO FRIENDS — COOLNESS
ABSOLUTELY NECESSARY TO SUCCESS

IT is true that the offensive and defensive
feats of *jiu-jitsu* combat may be undertaken
without any preliminary training. Yet it is
equally true that not so good results are secured by this course as are to be had when the
application of the work is based on a proper

foundation of well-trained muscles and with other parts of the body properly prepared for the tasks that are to be exacted of them.

Jiu-jitsu does not demand muscular development to the same extent that it is needed in the practice of boxing or of wrestling, but it is well—and very nearly absolutely essential—to possess nerves and muscles that are especially trained to respond with lightning-like swiftness to the demands that are put upon them by the peculiarities of the Japanese style of personal encounter.   The Japanese blows are struck with greater speed than are those used by Anglo-Saxon boxers, and must be landed with far greater exactness.

The expert at *jiu-jitsu* is able to defeat the boxer easily and signally.   It follows, therefore, that the blow must have both superior speed and effect.

What, then, are the methods of preliminary training that give these advantages.   It has been pointed out in my previous works on this subject that the Japanese experts themselves differ considerably as to the best methods of bringing the muscles and their governing nerves into the most serviceable condition. Just as *jiu-jitsu* has been made to evolve into at least a half-dozen distinct though closely related schools of execution, so there are many different ideas among the initiated as to how the body is to be prepared. Some teachers of *jiu-jitsu* give no preliminary gymnastic work, but proceed at once to the practice of the feats of attack and defence, and rely upon continued practice in this work to give the muscles the peculiar tone that is needed. Other teachers, again, have their own special systems of gymnastics, and these latter, while differing in form, are all based upon and meet the same requirements.

In the three volumes that the author has offered to the public on the subject of physical training according to Japanese methods there has been explained an eclectic system of preparation that is undoubtedly the best that Japan has to offer. This system is based, for the most part, on the teachings of one of the most modern of Tokio's *jiu-jitsu* experts, while features have been taken also from the teachings of many other noted exponents of to-day.

This system of bodily training, then, as described in the author's three preceding volumes,
furnishes the best muscular basis for the work
that is to be explained in this volume.　But,
once the muscles have been put in proper re-
sponsive condition, there are other demands to
be considered.　For instance, the Japanese
does not strike with his clenched fist, but with
the inner or little finger edge of the palm.
This edge of the palm, then, must be put in
the most favourable trim for severe attack.
The edge must be hard—capable of inflicting
injury and of enduring sharp concussion.

For training the edge of the hand thus there
is a very simple method that calls only for time
and patience.　Strike the edge of the hand
lightly but repeatedly against a wooden or
some similar surface.　It is never necessary to
increase the severity of this training blow, but
at least twenty minutes daily should be given
to this hardening process.　For this no time
need be taken from other occupations.　When
seated reading, exercise the edge of that hand
which is not employed in holding the book.
At times when neither hand is otherwise

occupied the edges of both may be exercised simultaneously. The importance of so training the edges of the hands is not to be estimated lightly, and this toughening should be followed diligently for some months. The harder the edge of the hand is made the more effective will be the blows struck with it, and with the least exertion on the part of the combatant.

At the same time the parts of the body that are likely to be struck by an opponent must be hardened. This is accomplished most effectively by daily assaults upon these parts of the body. In other words, harden any given part of the body by repeated endurance of the kind of *jiu-jitsu* attack that would be made upon it. This attack, when made in practice, is not employed with the same severity that would be used in actual, serious combat.

An attack against the solar plexus may be resisted, to some extent, by drawing in the abdomen and tensing its muscles; but this is not all-sufficient. The endurance of light but repeated attacks on the solar plexus will do far more to harden that sensitive spot against actual and vicious attack.

He who is to do well in the mastery of *jiu-jitsu* must have from the outset a friend with whom he can practise the work continuously and enthusiastically. This practice must be had daily, and must be carried on with as much severity as can be employed without inflicting injury of serious nature. A movement, when first undertaken, should be gone through with slowly and analytically. Just as soon as the idea has been mastered, then every energy should be devoted to performing the feat with ever increasing speed. In order to be effective in the end, one must be able to do all of the work with a speed resembling that of thought. Every time the beginner employs a given feat he must make it a point to carry it out with all the speed that is in him. Speed must become so much of a *habit* that, in the end, its employment will be automatic—without thought!

To the student of *jiu-jitsu* combat this bit of advice will be found excellent:

"Don't be in a hurry to show off a new trick to your friends."

Japanese combat is all so new and so wonderful to the Occidental beginner, and so superior in effectiveness to our own styles of encounter, that the learner is tempted to display his new acquirement just as soon as he thinks he has mastered it. Don't be like a boy with a new toy. Don't expect, after a few trials of a new feat, to be able to down a friend who is unfortunate enough to know nothing better than Anglo-Saxon methods of defence. The expert boxer has devoted years to the practice of his art. It is unreasonable to expect that, after merely an afternoon's practice, you will be able to defeat him at his own game. The beginner who disregards this advice, instead of proving his own impregnability, will go down to defeat and expose himself to ridicule.

Never allow yourself to become flustered. From the outset cultivate absolute coolness, or you will never become thoroughly proficient. If you discover any flaw in trick of attack or defence, take defeat philosophically; note just what the flaw is and study, patiently and calculatingly, how to remedy it. In the beginning it is well always to practise with the same friend. After a while try the work on other fellow students. Occasional change from one opponent to another is advisable in order to escape the danger of falling into a style of work too automatically conceived. When you have an opponent who always makes a given move in an exact and unvarying way you are in danger of falling into his rut, and thus of being unprepared to meet a slight variation in the performance of the feat.

As to the amount of practice needed for the perfect mastery of any one trick, this depends, in the first place, upon the nature of the trick, and much more upon the qualifications of the performer. Some feats are so simple that they have been mastered forever after a very few trials. Others will require frequent practice during a period of many weeks.

Be patient. Expect little or nothing in a hurry. Place an invariable exaction upon yourself that each given feat must be performed a little better each time that it is undertaken. Don't balk at repeated practice of each trick. Practice must be continued until the feat is performed with the utmost speed of which the body is capable. Even when this speed is obtained. practice must go patiently on until the

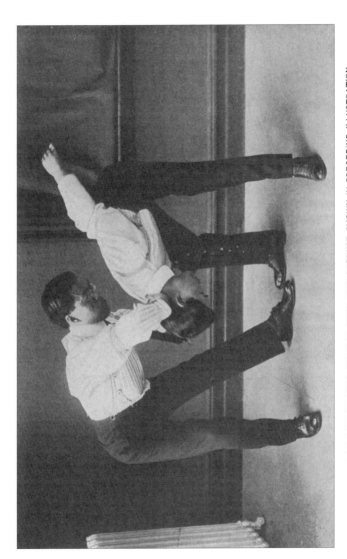

No. 2.   AN ADVANTAGE THAT RESULTS FROM THE DEFENSE SHOWN IN PRECEDING ILLUSTRATION.

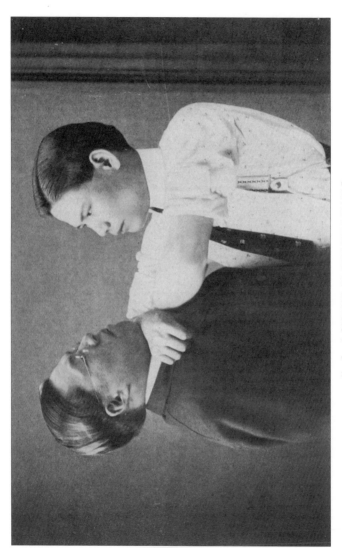

No. 3.   A CORRECT JIU-JITSU THROAT-HOLD.

student performs whatever trick is needed as a matter of second nature, and with the prompt response and the precision of an automaton.

The student who has but limited time for practice will do well not to attempt the mastery of all the feats described in this volume. A dozen tricks, well-mastered, will make any man formidable — invincible to an opponent who does not understand them. If a dozen tricks be taken up at the outset, and are acquired with perfection of detail and speed, then the student may add one or two, and one or two more, and so on, as he finds the time.

Good nature is highly necessary. Many of the blows, holds, and pressures of *jiu-jitsu* inflict considerable momentary pain, which is borne more easily when it is remembered that the other fellow is taking the same chances.

In the art of *jiu-jitsu* mere theory, valuable though it is, will not suffice. One may learn by rote all of the descriptions given in this volume and be hardly a whit better off in the moment of vicious assault upon his person. The student's motto must be practice—constant practice! It is worth something to be

able to walk abroad secure in the knowledge
that though one possesses but very ordinary
physique, he is the master of tricks of combat
that make him more than the physical peer of
an adversary who is much larger and stronger!

CHAPTER II

WHEN attacking an opponent men of all degrees of barbarity and of civilisation are prone to seize the intended victim by the throat. Nor is the reason for the popularity of this style of attack hard to find. It is hard to conceive of a man so ignorant that he does not know that, by shutting off his adversary's power of breathing, he thereby does away with the possibility of prolonged resistance.

So overmastering is a severe throat-hold that the victim, if he is an untrained man, rarely has the presence of mind to relieve himself of the oppression by a counter attack on some portion of his assailant's body. Instead, the victim involuntarily clutches at the oppressing hands that are choking off his supply of air.

and tries to drag them away.   If the strangling hold is well taken it is all but impossible to force the attacking hands away in time, and the victim is reduced to submission.

Evidently strangling was as popular among the primitive Japanese as it has been in other parts of the world, for the *jiu-jitsu* adepts of ancient Japan have handed down to us the results of much thought both as to the taking of strangle holds and the quick and efficient breaking of them.   There are many styles of throat attack and of defence from it, and in this volume enough of this work will be described to apply to any possible problem in connection with choking as a means of combat.

In Anglo-Saxon countries few men will be found who have progressed far in throat attack.   Almost invariably the attack is made merely by grasping the front of the throat with both hands and doing one's best to retain the hold until the opponent's resistance is stopped. Such a throat-hold is indicated in photograph No. 1.   It will be well to study the counter of the intended victim carefully, and to verify and acquire it by considerable patient practice.

The victim places his hands, with palms together, under the assailant's arms, and with backs of the hands outward. With a quick upward movement the victim thrusts his joined hands between the arms of his assailant. As soon as the victim's hands have gone upward as far as they will go the joined hands are separated, and each is thrown violently out far to its own side of the body.

If this is not wholly clear, take another look at the illustration. Imagine that the victim's hands are a little higher up, and that the outer sides of his upper arms press against the inner sides of his assailant's arms. Now, imagine the victim's hands to be shot out suddenly sideways with all the force possible. His moving arms strongly force away the arms of the attacking man, and the throat-hold is broken.

Where too much muscular strength is not needed for breaking the throat-hold this is the best method, and it is also the swiftest known to *jiu-jitsu*. Where more force is required, however, in order to break the assailant's grip, the method illustrated in the photograph opposite page 110 in my former work, *Japanese*

Physical Training, is needed.   This latter feat
is slower of execution, but supplies greater
force in breaking a throat-hold.   In this latter
feat the victim clenches his hands, with fingers
tightly interlaced, just before his abdomen.
Both arms are given a violent swing to the
left, up and over, striking the assailant's right
elbow and carrying away the attacking arms
by sheer force of momentum.

Returning to the defence shown in the first
illustration, where the victim shoots both hands
up *between* the assailant's arms, this feat can
be followed up by a very effective piece of work
that transforms the recent victim into the new
assailant.   It will be remembered that the late
victim's hands, by the time he has broken the
throat-hold, are in between the opponent's
arms.   From this position let the late victim,
without an instant's delay, throw his hands
around the back of the opponent's head, join-
ing the hands—and interlacing the fingers—
just at the base of the skull.   Jerk the opponent's head forward and downward toward
the ground.   It is easy to bear him down, and
at the same time the new assailant should dart

backward two or three steps, dragging his bent-over adversary with him and forcing him to the floor with a quick jerk, stretching the man prostrate and face downward.

But if the man whose head is caught in this unpleasant fashion is versed in *jiu-jitsu*, and is quick enough, it is possible for him to escape being thrown face downward, and to be ready at once to resume the aggressive. American physical trainers have assured me that there is next to no possibility of defence when this back-of-the-head hold is well taken. It has been my pleasure to show several of these gentlemen that they were in error.

Allow the companion with whom you are practising to secure this back-of-the-head hold and to bend your head as close to the floor as is shown in photograph No. 2. Make a slight feint of " ducking " and of wriggling your head out at the left. Almost unconsciously your assailant will throw his clasped hands over to the same side in order to prevent your escape. Follow this feint instantly by a decided " duck " and a wriggle-out at your right side, and you will escape and bring yourself erect. It must be remembered, however, to make the feint to the left not too pronounced, and to follow it up instantly by the more vigorous effort to the right. Of course, if preferred, the feint may be made to your right, and the escape to your left. Now, for a scientific *jiu-jitsu* throat-hold that is not broken easily. It will have to be performed slowly at first until the theory is mastered. Begin the attack by extending your hands palms upward. Force the hands under the opponent's coat-collar on either side of his neck, and with the fingers take a forcible grip of the collar on either side of the neck and well back. Now, twist the hands over to the inside so that the backs are up and the tips of the thumbs against the throat. At a point on either side just below the level of the "Adam's apple," and an inch or so back from its perpendicular line, press the balls of the thumbs severely in. This exact spot of contact for the thumbs can be found by experimenting on one's own throat until the place is located where the pressure accomplishes strangling most effectively.

Practise this feat over and over again until it

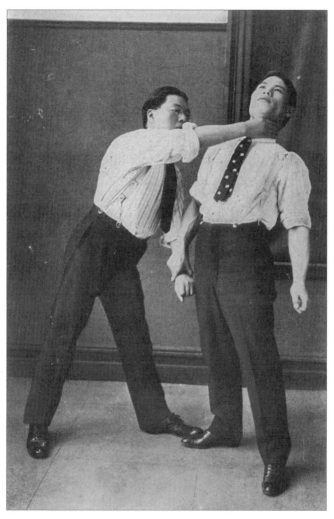

No. 4. SIMULTANEOUS ATTACK—THROAT-HOLD AND HAND-PINCH.

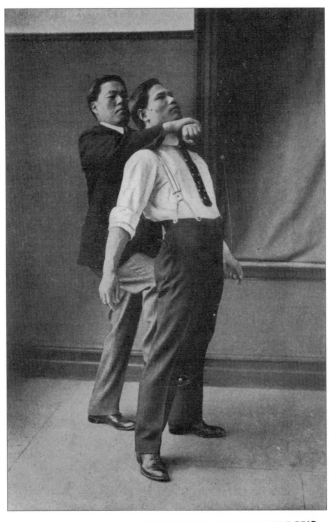

No. 5. A THROAT-HOLD AND THROW BY AN ASSAILANT IN THE REAR.

is possible to seize the opponent by the coat-collar and to apply the strangling pressure with the balls of the thumbs with great speed and effectiveness. It is all but impossible to break this hold when it is well taken, for the fingers grip the coat-collar so tightly as to make their dislodgment no easy task, and the balls of the thumbs accomplish the strangling with certainty.

Still another scientific throat-hold is depicted in photograph No. 3. Here the assailant's arms are crossed. With his left hand the attacking one grips the victim's left coat-collar well forward, and with his right hand grips the victim's right coat-collar—and further back on this side. With the grip of both hands tightly maintained the fists are drawn closer together across the front of the victim's throat, and in such manner that severe pressure with the assailant's right fore-arm is applied to the right side of the victim's throat just back of the "Adam's apple." With a little experimenting, a very effective strangling trick is secured, and one that cannot be defeated by either of the counters already described.

When employing either of these strangles the assailant can, if he wishes, strike one of his knees smartly into the crotch or abdomen of his victim, and thus bring the attack to a sharp culmination.   The victim, of course, if he be equally quick, can counter this last blow by raising one of his knees to block the attack.

For either of the two strangle-holds just described there is but one useful style of defence. It requires presence of mind and the quickest of action, and, for both reasons, this counter should be practised persistently, and always with all possible speed, until it becomes second nature, and is performed all but automatically. This style of defence calls for a solar-plexus jab.   Failing in touching the plexus, the attack may be delivered full in the abdomen and with emphatic force.   If this defence is well made the assailant may be depended upon to let go his throat-hold with alacrity.

The jab in the solar plexus is delivered with the points of the first and second fingers, and with the forefinger uppermost.   At the instant of striking the hand is turned quickly to the outside, so that not only is the blow delivered,

but a sickening "dig" accompanies the act.
If, however, the two fingers are struck against
the abdomen, the "dig" need not be added, as
it accomplishes little or nothing in this instance.

Naturally the question will arise:

"Why may not the blow be given as well
with the fist as with the tips of the two first
fingers?"

The answer to this query will be apparent
after a moment of thought. The blow with
the fist distributes the shock of impact over
too extensive a surface, and the effect is much
less than when the shock is confined to a very
small surface by striking with the tips of two
fingers. It is for the same reason that the
Japanese adept does not employ his clenched
fist against an adversary's bone, but always
uses the little finger edge of his palm to admin-
ister a sharp blow.

Patient study should be given to the few
feats of attack and defence described in this
chapter, and this remark applies with equal
force to all of the feats that are to follow.
First of all, grasp the idea, and then perfect
theory by slow, analytical practice. Once the

theory has been mastered, work for gradually increasing speed until, at last, it is possible to perform the feat with the utmost quickness and with never a fumble. Much depends upon thorough acquirement of the theory, and as much more depends on slowly and studiously increasing the speed until it has reached the limit of quick performance.

Nothing is gained by hasty and careless study of *jiu-jitsu* work. He who takes it up in this slip-shod manner will find that he has added little or nothing to his expertness in personal encounter.

BE THOROUGH—PATIENT—PAINSTAKING!

CHAPTER III

IN addition to the throat-hold throw-offs
already described there is one that must be
acquired by every *jiu-jitsian*. This feat may
be designated as the "cork-screw throw-off,"
or may be known by any more fanciful name
that suits the pleasure of the student.

Suppose that the assailant has employed his
right hand in securing a throat-hold on the
victim, or in forcing his hand under the chin;
and that the assailant's left arm is thrown
around the lower back of the victim. Such an
attack is shown in the illustration opposite
page 104 of *Japanese Physical Training*. It
is in this case that the victim may employ
the "cork-screw throw-off" to very good
advantage.

This is done by the victim throwing up his left arm inside his opponent's right. On the inside the victim's arm crosses the fore-arm of the assailant. Now, the victim's arm is forced out over the outside of the assailant's, the two engaged arms of the combatants crossing at about the elbow. Now, the victim's arm, on the outside of the assailant's, is forced in under the latter's upper arm, so that the backs of the victim's fingers press hard against the upper ribs of the assailant.

It is important that this position be studied until it has been obtained to perfection. As soon as the position has been taken correctly, the victim should tense his own arm in such a way as to crush and weaken his adversary's, the victim at the same time giving as hard a dig as he can with the backs of his left fingers against the assailant's ribs. At the same time the victim forces his right hand under the assailant's chin, the thumb on one side of the throat and the fingers on the other. And the assailant's head is forced as far as possible over backward or sideways. In this manner a complete throw-off of the assailant's attack is made.

It will serve for the student to remember
that he has not mastered this feat in all its details until he is able to throw off the attack in-
fallibly.   Once the principle of the thing has
been mastered, all future effort should be
directed to gaining speed in the performance.
It is not a difficult trick to acquire, and it is
very effective.   Should the assailant employ
both hands in attacking the throat, then the
victim must employ both of his arms against
those of his adversary in the "cork-screw
throw-off," and it is in this double style of the
work that the effectiveness of the throw-off is
most quickly seen.

In photograph No. 4 is shown an attack and
defence so quickly executed as to appear to be
a simultaneous attack.   The assailant has secured the victim's throat with the right hand,
but the victim has caught the left hand with a
pinch.   This pinch is inflicted by pressing the
ball of the thumb into the back of the hand
between the bases of the little finger and its
neighbour.   The thumb is pressed in heavily,
and ground over the muscles and nerves en-
countered there.   It will be seen that the vic-

tim, thanks to his quickness, has secured rather the best of it; for, while both of the assailant's hands are now engaged, the victim has his left hand free for whatever style of attack seems best suited, supposably a solar-plexus jab. Under these circumstances it will be best for the assailant to free his captured hand, if he can do so by a quick wrench, and to follow up this unsuccessful attack by one more accurately judged.

In photograph No. 5 is shown a style of throat-attack that is made from behind. The assailant is simultaneously raising one knee to give a severe blow in the buttocks or at the base of the spine. The knee-blow may be given, if preferred, against either kidney, the point of striking being in the soft part under the last rib. There is a third movement in this attack, which consists of dragging the victim over and dropping him on his back. All three movements should be performed as nearly simultaneously as possible.

This may all be done so swiftly that it would seem impossible to devise an effective counter for the protection of the victim, but the Japan-

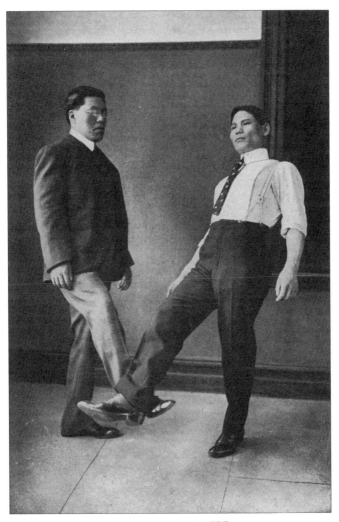

No. 6. THE WRONG WAY TO TRIP.

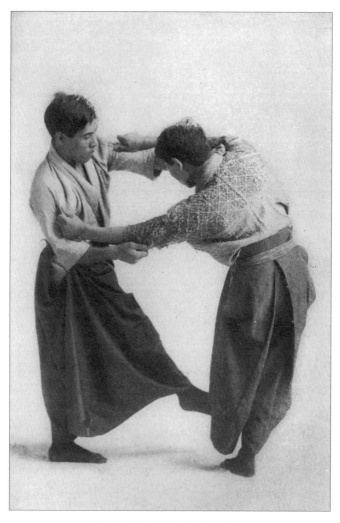

No. 7. THE RIGHT WAY TO TRIP.

ese have solved the difficult problem.   It will be understood, of course, that the defence must be made with great speed.

The simplest defence consists, for the victim, in bending the body over to the right with a swift twist, giving the victim an opportunity to jab his left elbow backward with force into the assailant's solar plexus or abdomen, the force of this shock causing the assailant to abandon his hold.   This will do well enough for the beginner in *jiu-jitsu*, but in the meantime he should carefully prepare for the two forms of defence that are now to be described.

At the instant of attack the victim seizes his adversary's wrist with his own left hand.   On the inside of the arm, about an inch above the elbow joint, and in line with the "knob" of bone at the joint is a nerve that may be severely pressed with the end of the thumb with a great deal of resulting pain.   The victim's right hand is thrown around the assailant's arm at this point, from the outside, and the thumb is pressed forcibly against the nerve.   The student should devote considerable study to the location and punishment of this nerve.

Now, the victim, with his left hand around
his opponent's right wrist and his right hand
attacking the nerve above the assailant's right
elbow, breaks the assailant's hold, forcing the
latter's right arm up over the victim's head and
down again, so that the victim has squirmed to
the right of this attacking arm.   In the next
breath the victim throws his own right thigh
back of his assailant's right thigh.   The victim's left arm goes around the back of his assailant, while the victim's right hand is thrown
across the front of the assailant's body, down,
outside, a᾽ d back of the assailant's left knee,
back of which it hooks.   Now, by giving a
quick wrench forward and upward at the assailant's left knee, the victim is able to drop
his opponent to the floor.

The other form of defence consists in bringing the assailant's right arm forward over the
right shoulder, after the manner illustrated in
photograph No. 24.   This is done at the instant when the assailant's hands are forced
apart in the manner just described.   The palm
of the assailant's captured hand is held upward,
while the victim pulls down severely at the

wrist, forcing the assailant's arm bones to "go the wrong way," and thus inflicting more pain than can be borne with composure. The pressure must be severe enough to force the balked assailant to surrender, and the pressure can be made hard enough, as will be readily understood, to break the assailant's captured arm.

In performing this feat the student must be urged to locate the mentioned nerve above the elbow so thoroughly that he can attack it without a second's hesitation or fumbling. And when the assailant's arm is brought over the shoulder the palm of the hand must be up; if the palm is held down it will be understood that the captured arm will bend readily, and the victim's defence will thus be rendered worthless. And while above, it is suggested that the assailant's captured arm be brought over the right shoulder, it is even better if the manœuvre be so made that the arm is brought, instead, over the victim's left shoulder, and for a reason that will be comprehended after another study of photograph No. 24. But the defence of the victim must be made so quickly that circumstances decide which shoulder of the victim is to be used.

In Chapter I. reference has been made to the fact that the *jiu-jitsian* does not employ his clenched fist in striking a blow, but uses the edge of his hand, generally the little finger edge. This does not mean *the edge of the little finger*, which should never be struck, but the edge of the palm on the little finger side. In striking, sometimes the palm of the hand is turned upward, and sometimes downward, just as the nature of the blow requires for striking most severely. In some instances, as in striking upward under the chin, the thumb edge of the palm is used, the thumb being folded downward over the palm.

Here is a list of the more important blows that may be struck with the edge of the hand:

Lower Leg.—Across the shin on either side, and well to the front; strike half-way up the lower leg.

Upper Leg.—Strike half-way between knee and trunk, either across front of leg, or at outside of leg somewhat to the front.

Side Blow.—Squarely on either side of the

lower trunk, in the soft part just below the last rib.

Kidney.—Strike over this organ in small of back, in soft part just below last rib.

Wrist.—On either side, just back of joint.

Fore-arm.—On either side, half-way between wrist and elbow.

Upper Arm.—Strike across front of biceps, or on outside of arm and well to the front; in either case point of striking to be midway between elbow and shoulder.

Collar-bone.—In a close clinch, open at one side, strike with little finger edge of palm, hand almost perpendicular and fingers pointing up, on collar-bone midway between breast-bone and point of shoulder. (Too sharp a blow will fracture this bone.)

Shoulder.—A sharp downward blow on top of shoulder, midway between neck and point of shoulder. (A blow that causes a good deal of pain and subsequent soreness.)

Side of the Neck.—Midway between jaw-bone and collar-bone.

Back of the Neck.—Too dangerous. Do not employ, except in a case of "life or death."

Instead, when striking from behind, use heel of hand, fingers pointing upward. Strike heel of hand just at the base of the skull, with a combined forward and upward movement. And even this blow is hardly less dangerous. Both blows are mentioned more by way of caution that they be avoided by the experimenting student.

Blow across Base of Spine.—Too dangerous. Instead, employ blow over kidney.

All of the blows struck with the edge of the hand are given smartly and with a good deal of force. In striking at throat or neck the right hand of assailant is used against the victim on his right side, instead of at his left, in order that the blow may be given more force.

The edge of the hand should not be struck across the "Adam's apple," but the edge of the fore-arm, covered by the coat-sleeve, may be employed for striking here when necessary.

CHAPTER IV

THE RIGHT WAY AND THE WRONG WAY TO
TRIP AN OPPONENT—HOW TO DODGE THE
TRIP — HOW TO KNEEL AND TRIP AN
ADVERSARY —"COUNTERS" THAT ARE
POSSIBLE

TRIPPING is so general a trick among all
the peoples that develop the art of personal combat as to seem to call for but scant
mention.   Yet in this country there are so
many who do not know how to trip correctly
that some hints are needful.   In *jiu-jitsu* the
trip is an element of prime importance.

In a trip that is delivered while the assailant
is standing, the right foot is always employed
against the adversary's left, and the left against
the adversary's right.   Right foot is never employed against right foot, nor left against left.

In a trip that the assailant delivers from a
kneeling position, on the contrary, it is the
right foot that is employed against the victim's
right, and the left against the victim's left.

In tripping the collar-and-elbow grip is the favourite among *jiu-jitsians*. Yet one hand may seize the coat or shirt close to the arm. Suppose it is desired to throw an opponent at your own left side. With your arms swing him around to your left, forcing him to travel at least a third of a circle. If this is done swiftly and effectively it will leave the victim standing on his right foot, with his left clear of the ground for an instant. In that instant apply your left foot to his right —his sole prop —and knock it from under him, sending him to the ground.

As to the method of kicking a foot from under the victim, the kick is always delivered against the outside of his foot. The assailant's foot moves swiftly over the ground, leaving it just a hair's-breadth at the instant of impact. The greatest force of the kick is delivered just at the ankle bone. Thus the pain caused the victim adds its effect to that of the impetus given by the kick, and the throw is all the more easily made. For it is human nature, when a foot is pained by a kick, to lift, or partly to lift, that foot from the ground. This is an

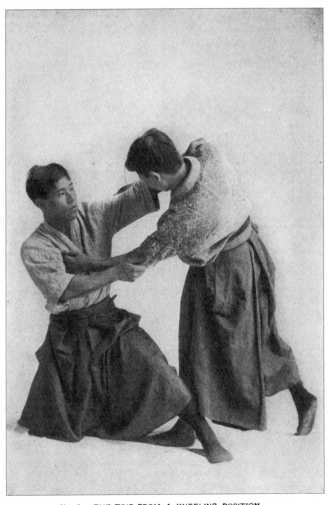

No. 8. THE TRIP FROM A KNEELING POSITION.

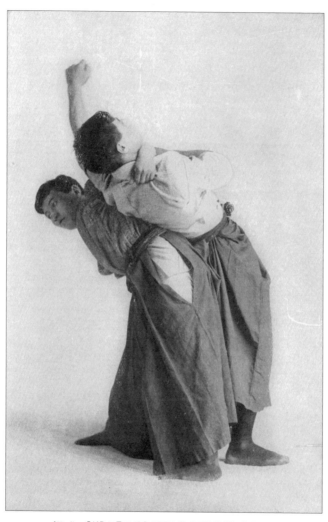

No. 9   THROAT-HOLD WITH THROW OVER THE HIP.

application of a well-known fact that is worthy of the wily Oriental.

It is to be observed that, in tripping under the most favourable circumstances, only the foot that is to be kicked is to be on the ground, the other being in the air, *and the victim's body bent well over to the side to which he is to be thrown.*

The only feasible counter to this trip is to get the other foot from the air to the ground in time, and to regain as nearly erect position as possible. Yet even with both feet of the victim on the ground it is often possible to throw him by this trip. At the moment of impact between the assailant's foot and the victim's the victim's trunk is drawn violently to the side to which it is desired to throw him.

When both of the victim's feet are on the ground a simple counter to the assailant's trip is possible. Just as the assailant goes to kick the victim should dexterously draw back the threatened foot and succeed in striking the assailant's engaged foot *at the outside*—in other words, delivering the same style of kick that was intended for himself.

If the opponent is instructed and is wary it is often necessary for the assailant to swing his man around in a part circle two or three times before the tripping kick can be delivered with the proper effect. These continuous swing-arounds should be made at least three or four times in the same direction; then, if the assailant thinks it will be to his advantage, he may swiftly reverse the direction of the swing. Often, by so doing, he will catch his intended victim off guard and have an easy victory.

Photographs Nos. 6 and 7 illustrate graphically the wrong and the right methods of delivering the kick in tripping. In the first illustration it will be noted that both adversaries have their right feet engaged. In the second illustration the assailant is employing his right foot in a kick against his adversary's left.

Sometimes it is found so difficult to catch the intended victim off his guard in a standing trip that the kneeling trip is resorted to by the assailant. In this case the combatant making the assault takes a catch-as-catch-can hold and drops to one knee, thrusting the other foot out before him. Over the lower half of this extended leg the assailant swings his adversary and accomplishes the throw. The trick is performed with ease after a little practice. The kneeling trip has this decided advantage: That the assailant is closer to his victim at the moment of the fall, and is able more promptly to apply any advisable tactics for reducing the victim to complete submission. Some of these methods of following up the advantage secured by a throw will be described in the following chapter.

In the kneeling trip it will be noted, with care, that the right leg is employed against the right, the left against the left. The relative positions of the two combatants are accurately shown in photograph No. 8.

There is a very simple and convincing feat that can be employed in many an emergency of combat, and it can be ended, if desired, in a trip. While standing at the opponent's left seize his left wrist with the right hand. It is important to hold the back of the victim's wrist outward, with the little finger edge of the captured hand downward. Have your own thumb against the under edge of the captured wrist, the fingers gripping tightly over the upper edge. With your left hand seize the open fingers of the victim's captured hand. Bend the fingers relentlessly backward as if trying to make them touch the back of the victim's fore-arm. Of course it will hurt him, and the result will be that the assailant is able to swing his victim around and around to the left as long as is desired, and all the while the victim is suffering from the pain in his captured wrist and fingers, and is unable to resist.

But it is a better plan, after having secured the hold, and after having started to bend the captured fingers backward, to shoot both of your arms out ahead of you and to hold them out rigidly, thus forcing the victim away from you while continuing to hurt him, and forcing him to run along ahead of you. In this way he is prevented from making any countering use with the free hand at his other side.

This description should be studied carefully, and every detail of the directions followed closely in actual practice until the feat is thoroughly mastered. By the time that it is thoroughly understood it will be possible for the assailant to seize the victim's wrist and fingers and to begin to apply the pressure all in the space of a fleeting instant. Speed counts for almost everything in securing the hold and beginning the excruciating pressure on the fingers.

If it is desired to throw the adversary, seize his left wrist and fingers and apply the backward pressure in the same manner. At the same time bend slightly and make a half turn to the left, placing yourself in front of your victim, with your buttocks toward his right side, and your left buttock against his middle. Now twist his captured arm well around to the left, swinging your own body somewhat to the left at the same time, and, by the pull on his captured arm, accomplish a throw over your right buttock.

This throws the victim down on his right side. Instantly step squarely on his right fore-arm, pinning it to the ground. You still have hold of his left wrist and left fingers. Holding his captured wrist firmly, continue to bend his captured fingers over backward, keeping up the painful pressure until he surrenders.

Now comes a separate feat that has a bearing upon the one just described. Facing the victim, seize his left wrist with your right hand, and force his arm up. At the same instant seize him at the inner bend of his left elbow with your left hand, using this elbow clutch also to assist in raising his arm. This arm should be forced to a little above horizontal position, sideways.

Having secured this hold, swing around under the captured arm, having your back to the victim's left side as you pass him to go to his rear, and complete the turn by facing the same way that he does as you get behind him. Force his captured hand as far up his back as you can, holding it there with your right hand. Force his captured elbow as far across his back as you can by the aid of your left hand, with which you have all the while held his elbow. The victim's hand can be forced so far up behind his back as to cause him a great deal of pain, and by closing up to him you can hold his arm locked at your pleasure.

Now, in the feat described before this one, the victim, if he is initiated, can prevent having his fingers bent backward if he tightly clenches his fist at the instant when his wrist is seized. But, in that case the assailant, having the wrist already captured, can employ his left hand in seizing the victim's elbow, passing under the arm and locking the victim's arm behind him in the manner just detailed.

Here again the victim can interpose an effective block by side-stepping with his foot to the left just as the assailant is passing under his arm, and the assailant will trip himself and fall to the ground. But the assailant should be watching for this snare, and, if he sees his antagonist's foot extended to trip him, the assailant should stop short. But the assailant has an effective move left. His left elbow is just in position to give the victim an effective jab in the short ribs. This elbow jab can be given so severely as to incapacitate the victim.

CHAPTER V

THERE is a throat-hold, with an accompanying throw, that is very much used by
the Japanese. When attempted by the expert
this feat is easily and successfully performed,
but it requires considerable practice, and the
neophyte must not look for immediate skill
with this trick.

An excellent idea of the manner of taking
the tackle may be gained from photograph
No. 9. Indeed, nearly everything except the
actual fall is clearly shown.

The victim has been attacked at his left side.
The assailant has thrown his left arm under
his victim's left arm, the assaulting arm passing
squarely over the victim's throat, and the hand

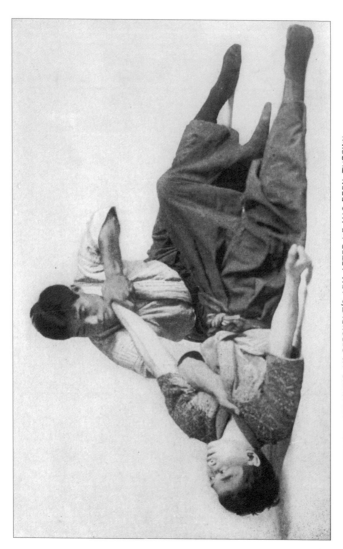

No. 10. STRAINING AN OPPONENT'S ARM AFTER HE HAS BEEN THROWN.

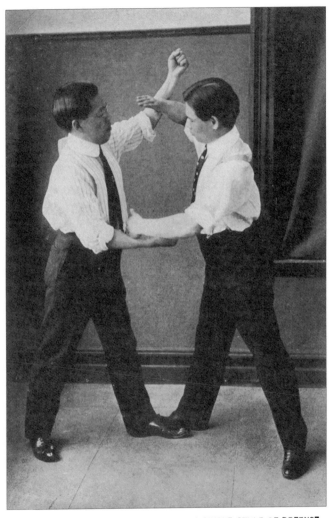

No. 11. JIU-JITSU AGAINST THE BOXER—A SIMPLE STYLE OF DEFENSE.

being clutched in the garment just back of the right shoulder. At the same time the assailant has so placed himself that his buttocks are against those of the victim. The assailant having bent forward, all that remains is a quick throw over the hip.

Were it not for one thing, this hold would be, in itself, sufficiently disconcerting to the victim. But the latter has his right hand free, and, if he be merely held in this position, he could use the free hand for mischief. From the nature of their relative positions all that is to be left to the assailant by way of making his attack final is to complete the throw over the hip and leave his adversary prostrate. One with ordinary muscular development can readily acquire the knack of combining his pull with a quick wrench of the body that accomplishes the fall. Speed in securing the hold is not difficult of attainment. The combination of hold and throw, performed so rapidly that the victim is on his back seemingly in a second from the instant when he is first attacked, is what calls for a good deal of practice. At the outset it is an excellent idea for the student to practise the hold and the throw separately—that is, so far as the performance with speed is concerned. Devote a certain number of trials to securing the hold as quickly as it can be done, then making a little pause before trying the throw. After that, make a few attempts in which the hold is taken in a leisurely way, followed by a throw as rapid as it can be made. By degrees the embryo *jiu-jitsian* will find speed in the entirety of the performance coming to him.

The feat known to Anglo-Saxon wrestlers as the "flying mare" is common to the Japanese, but is not looked upon as a performance of especial value. One that answers the purpose much better, when the muscular strength and the agility of the assailant are equal to the occasion, is the following:

Seize the wrist of the intended victim, and pull his captured arm over your shoulder from behind. In the same moment of doing this sink to the floor on the knee of the same side of the body as the shoulder over which the throw is being made. Retaining the hold on the victim's captured wrist with both hands.

force his hand straight downward until it touches, or nearly touches, the floor before you.

As soon as the victim's captured wrist has been forced as close to the floor as possible, rise quickly to your feet, bending your body backward in rising. This rise must be accomplished with such a movement of your own body that the victim will fall forward over the shoulder as you rise. He will land on the floor, and with this advantage—that you have retained your hold on his captured wrist, and that arm is at your mercy. It is possible, often, to step on his other arm, thus pinning it to the floor. There is nothing left that the victim can do, as your feet are too near his head for him to succeed in kicking you. Now, in bringing the victim's arm over the shoulder, there must be an invariable rule: If it is his left wrist that is seized, carry it over the right shoulder; if the right wrist is seized carry it over the left shoulder. If the right wrist, for instance, were carried over the right shoulder, then the intended victim would be squarely behind his assailant, and could throw his left arm around his adversary's neck and prevent the fall. But with the right arm carried over the left shoulder, the victim's left arm is kept out of the sphere of action and cannot be used in time to prevent the success of the assault.

At first, in training, it will be sufficient to make this throw slowly, relying upon each succeeding bit of practice to make the speed increase gradually. Even if the muscular strength is not at first adequate to the demands made upon it by this throw, repeated practice will bring about the needed muscular conditions by degrees.

Once the victim has been sent to the ground, what to do with him there, in order to prevent him from at once renewing the contest, becomes a matter of prime importance. It has been pointed out that some of the throws leave the victim in such a position that one of his arms may be secured by retaining the hold taken upon it at the beginning of the throw, while the other arm may be stepped upon. In cases where the defeated combatant falls so that he lies over one of his arms, thus preventing stepping upon it, the assailant has the other

course open of stepping on his fallen adversary's side.

Photograph No. 10 depicts an excellent way
of reducing the victim to instant and complete
submission.   Here the assailant has fallen upon
his adversary in such manner that the former's
knee is pressing severely into the "soft part "
just below the last rib.   The assailant has retained his hold on the victim's left wrist, and
now draws that arm over his knee.   The inside
of the wrist is kept upward, and the downward
pressure at the wrist is such as to cause intense
pain in this captured arm.

It is imperative that this position of the
wrist of the captured arm be thoroughly
understood.   With the wrist up and the arm
being pressed severely downward the arm is
being forced to bend in the way that Nature
did not intend it to bend.   In other words, the
assailant is trying to make the arm "bend the
wrong way," and it is apparent at first thought
that this process cannot be carried very far
without causing the most intense pain.   Indeed, if this backward pressure of the arm
across the knee be applied with too great

severity, the captured arm will be broken. **It** is sufficient, however, to give pressure enough to cause the victim to wince and surrender. The pain will disappear as soon as the pressure is abandoned—in case, of course, the pressure has not been applied so viciously as to break the bone.

It is to be noted, also, that the assailant has his knee under the captured arm at a point above the elbow. If the knee pressure were applied as far down as the back of the *fore-arm* there would not be leverage enough to cause the victim any appreciable pain.

So important is this principle, in many applications in *jiu-jitsu*, that it is well to repeat it in other words:

ALWAYS BEAR IN MIND, WHEN ATTEMPTING TO CAUSE PAIN IN THE ARM BY THIS TRICK, THAT THE ARM MUST BE FORCED BACKWARD IN THE WAY THAT NATURE DID NOT INTEND IT TO GO, AND THAT COUNTER-PRESSURE MUST BE APPLIED TO THE BACK OF THE UPPER ARM. IF THE ARM IS BENT IN THE DIRECTION THAT NATURE INTENDED IT TO BEND NO PAIN WILL BE CAUSED.

It will be noted also in photograph No. 10 that the assailant's right hand is well employed. The fingers of the hand are thrust inside the shirt, while the thumb is gripped outside. (This application of the hand to the lapel of a coat will answer the same purpose.)   The knuckles of the back of the assailant's hand are pressed with grinding force against the upper ribs of the victim at a point close to the shoulder.   The grip of the hand on the shirt or coat lapel gives leverage for more severe pressure of knuckles against ribs.   A little experimenting by the student upon himself will show that pressure of knuckles against the ribs at this point is productive of considerable pain. The victim in the case shown in photograph No. 10, being inflicted with severe pain at two points, and being at the same time incapable of countering, is quickly reduced to submission.

There are many applications of the principle of bending the arm in the wrong way that the student can discover by intelligent practice.   A few hints along this line will be given here.

With your right hand seize the victim's left wrist, and raise his arm horizontally sideways.

At the same time place the heel of the left hand under his upper arm, with the fingers upward across the back of the arm. Pull your right hand toward you, and push your left hand forcibly away from you. The victim's arm is made to go "the wrong way," and he can be forced to spin around as rapidly as his assailant can run around with him. The same feat may be performed by hooking the left fore-arm back of the victim's upper left arm and forcing back with your right hand at his wrist as before.

Or, coming up behind your victim, seize his upper arm at the back with one hand and push forward against his arm held horizontally, while with the other hand pulling backward on his wrist.

If the victim has been thrown forward on his face, fall so that one knee pins him down in the back. With the other knee resting squarely on the back of his arm, about midway between shoulder and elbow, pull the wrist upward. Simply the pressure of the knee across the back of his arm, augmented by the weight of the assailant above, is enough to cause a good deal

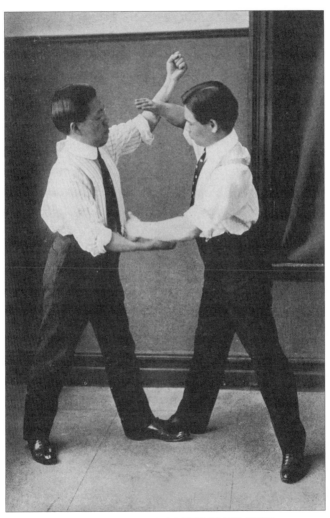

No. 12. DEFENSE AGAINST BOTH FISTS OF THE BOXER.

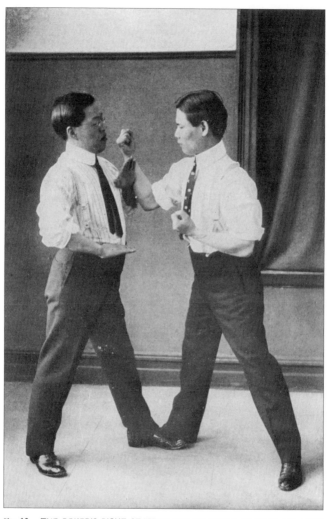

No. 13. THE BOXER'S RIGHT STOPPED AND ON GUARD AGAINST HIS **LEFT.**

of pain, but when to this downward pressure
of the knee is added the pulling up of the arm
at the wrist, the pain is such that the victim
cannot endure it.

CHAPTER VI

IT is difficult for the skilled boxer of the Anglo-Saxon race to realise that his pains-takingly acquired art is of no avail against the adept in *jiu-jitsu*. Yet the sooner this is realised to be a fact the sooner we shall cease reading in the newspapers of occasional in-stances where big Caucasians have tried pugil-ism on small Japanese, and have gone down ingloriously in the effort.

At least two or three times in every year we read of some Japanese who has had an altercation with an American policeman and has promptly put the latter on his back. Reinforcements, and still more reinforcements were called for before the Japanese was subdued and made a prisoner.

Last spring, in the Harvard gymnasium, there was an interesting encounter between Tyng, the strong man of that University, and a diminutive Japanese, a fellow student. Tyng tried his best foot-ball tackle, and threw his smaller opponent. But, after that, the Japanese eluded each effort to seize him. After the sport of dodging had continued for some time the Japanese darted in, took a lightning hold, and put Mr. Tyng upon the floor.

In Japanese ports a solitary native policeman has been known often to subdue as many as four turbulent sailors ashore from an American or English naval vessel, and to take the whole lot in submission to the police station. Indeed, the first American sailors to spend leave on shore in Japan after Perry had concluded the treaty with that country came home with the most wonderful tales. These sailors had had the not unusual lot to become involved in trouble ashore. They resorted to boxing with the natives. Upon their arrival here these same sailors declared that the country was peopled with devils whom the white man's best blows could not touch. Not only were these Japanese "devils" invulnerable to blows, but they actually picked up our men, one after another, and threw them into the sea!

Within the past year many exhibitions of *jiu-jitsu* have been given in the United States, and our younger athletes have had abundant opportunity to see *jiu-jitsu* and boxing contrasted. The result has been that these convinced athletes have started in promptly to acquire the Japanese art of meeting the boxer.

Seldom does the Japanese use his clenched fist. It is not considered "scientific." There is, of course, the legend of the Greek boxer who knew that he could deprive his adversary of his wind by a fist-blow in the abdomen, but who found that by driving the tips of his fingers against the abdomen he was able to penetrate deeply into the viscera. But the Japanese discovered, centuries ago, that the edge of the hand is not only more effective in warding off a blow, but that impact from such a blow will leave the adversary's muscles and bones aching. All of the common blows with the edge of the hand have been described in Chapter III.

Photograph No. 11 shows a *jiu-jitsian* in the act of warding off a left-hander from his adversary. Here the man on the defensive has not struck with the edge of his hand, but with the edge of his fore-arm just back of the wrist. This is as it happens, it being impossible to gauge exactly in the swift movement of defence. But the blow with the edge of the fore-arm is scarcely less formidable than that with the edge of the hand. It will be noted that the assailant is met with a blow against the middle of his own fore-arm.

This method of defence meets all requirements. In the first place it is effective as a ward-off. In the next place the defensive blow on the assailant's arm results in soreness of that member for the boxer, and will weaken the force of any subsequent blow that he may aim with it. The edges of the *jiu-jitsian's* hand and fore-arm are so hardened by constant practice that he suffers no pain from the impact. Note, also, in the illustration that the man on the defensive has his left hand in readiness to guard himself against the boxer's right.

Very often the boxer follows up his left with his right so rapidly that the two fists seem to shoot out simultaneously. Even in this case the *jiu-jitsian* is not caught unawares. His hands fly to encounter the boxer's arms, and the latter, baffled in this quick attack, has also some pain to take up his attention. (See photograph No. 12.) At the same time the boxer is apt to be convinced of the futility of trying to reach such an opponent.

And this style of defensive work is most readily acquired. After a very few bouts of practice the *jiu-jitsu* novice finds that he is able, if he is as quick as the boxer, to stop any and all blows much more easily than he could if trained only in boxing. Much depends, of course, on the hardness of the edge of the hand, but the way to secure this has been explained in Chapter III. It requires more time, however, to harden the edge of the hand properly than it does to learn defence with it.

A study of photograph No. 13 will result in a knowledge of how blows may be met by a defence close to the body. In this case the assailant is striking with a good deal of vigour, but the hand of the man on the defensive is forced to yield but little, and the blow is stopped.

At all times in practice, as in actual encounter, it is to be remembered that the *jiu-jitsian*, while warding off with one hand, is ever watchful and unceasingly ready to employ the edge of his other hand. This state of readiness does not call for one whit more of alertness or of agility in the *jiu-jitsian* than it does in the boxer. Any man who is quick enough to learn to box is quick enough to acquire the superior methods of *jiu-jitsu*.

In one defensive blow the heel of the hand is used with effect. This is in parrying by striking the outer bend of the boxer's elbow. The blow is struck in a combination of forward and upward movement, and with a good deal of smartness. This ward-off, when employed after much practice, is very effective, for, besides defending, it shakes the boxer's confidence in his ability to land a blow.

And in at least one form the heel of the hand is used in an aggressive blow. At the first sight of an opportunity the *jiu-jitsian* strikes swiftly and forcibly upward, landing the heel of his hand under the point of his adversary's chin. It is not difficult to register this blow, and this feat of à second's duration usually is enough to wind up the bout or fight.

At close quarters, with a clinch at one side, but where one combatant has his hand free at the other side, the edge of the free hand is struck against the collar-bone at about its middle. Struck even lightly, this blow causes pain. When the blow is delivered with full force it results in a fractured collar-bone. A little practice, beginning with very light blows, increasing gradually in severity, will give the student a fair idea of how hard a blow of this sort may be struck without breaking the bone. And, in accordance with the well-known rule that use hardens, the collar-bone may be strengthened very considerably by undergoing endurable assaults upon it.

Blows with the tips of the fingers—jabs—are never to be delivered against any portion of

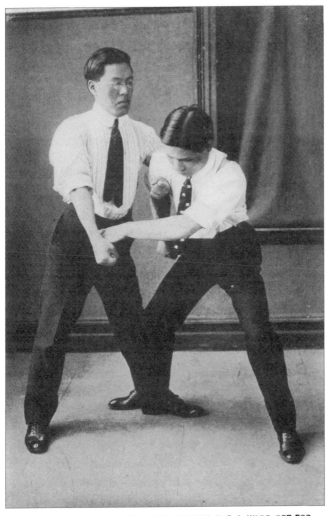

No. 14.   A HOOK OVER A LOW LEFT-HANDER AND A WARD-OFF FOR
THE RIGHT.

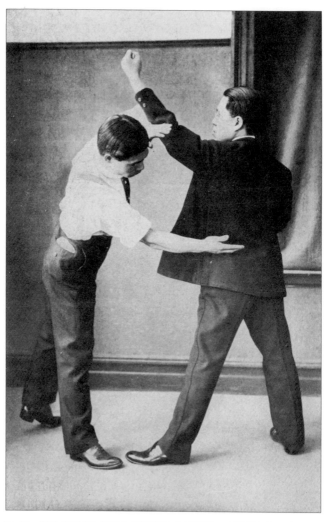

No. 15. THE KIDNEY BLOW AGAINST A BOXER — USEFUL UNDER MANY
OTHER CONDITIONS.

the body except the abdomen and the solar
plexus. A finger-tip blow against the ribs
will leave soreness there, but the concussion is
liable also to put the assailant's hand in bad
shape.

When striking up the arm of an adversary by
means of an edge-of-the-hand blow, the *jiu-
jitsian* is advised to practise the trick of forcing up his opponent's arm higher and darting
in under it to strike a blow of attack with the
edge of his unoccupied hand.

The best defensive trick of all, of course, is
one that stops the fight at the outset. The
writer will now describe a trick that he saw
performed in earnest, the defensive blow being
struck with full force. The assailant struck
out with his left fist. Quick as a flash the man
on the defensive side-stepped once to his own
left. In the same twinkling instant he let his
right hand fly upward, the edge of the hand
striking squarely across the assailant's right
jugular, at a point midway between the jaw
and the collar-bone.

A queer, gurgling sound came from the
throat of the stricken one. His knees gave

way under him, and he began to fall forward. Recovering, he succeeded in falling backward on his left hand and buttock. Less than half dazed, he was about to spring to his feet when his opponent's sharp warning came:

"Don't get up until I tell you to. If you do, you 'll get hurt!"

The defeated assailant obeyed, sinking back to the sidewalk, while the man who had defended himself drawled:

"After this you would better not go around hunting for trouble until you 've learned something about fighting. If you do, some day you will surely be hurt. Now, if you think you can go on and attend to your own affairs, you may get up and try it."

The assailant took the hint. So quickly and precisely had the defensive blow been given that it is doubtful if he understood just how his discomfiture had been brought about. And the best of it was that the man who had sought to provoke a fight had been stopped without sustaining any injury or disfigurement.

CHAPTER VII

TWO simple English words define a rule
without the observance of which no one
can expect to become anything like expert in
jiu-jitsu. These two words are:

Constant practice !

In taking up the ancient Japanese art of
attack and defence, many Anglo-Saxons will
be all enthusiasm at the outset, but will become gradually impatient under the monotony
of practising the feats so constantly that expertness comes as a matter of course.

There are those who will read these chapters,
and acquire a smattering knowledge of how

many of the feats are executed. Here, or close to this point, the study of some readers will stop. The little knowledge that has been absorbed will be laid by in a corner of the mind, to be called into active use only if the moment of need arrives. And then, in a possible crisis, the knowledge that has been so slightingly obtained will prove useless. Readers who study *jiu-jitsu* in this fashion will never become *jiu-jitsians*.

"I know how *that* is done," reflects some reader, after he has gone over the description and has scanned an illustration; he practises the thing a few times with a friend—and then the feat is learned and the knowledge is ready for use!

Any reader who is satisfied to acquire his knowledge of the Japanese art so easily would do better to save his time at the outset by devoting it to some study to which he will be more faithful.

The few descriptions given in the last chapter would seem to indicate very easy mastery of that part of the subject. All that was written can be read thoughtfully in a half an hour; in another half-hour each of the feats can be practised several times with a complaisant friend—and the thing seems simple and easy enough! Many readers will be surprised when they are told that even the few feats explained in the last chapter should be practised assidu ously for several weeks.

Yet this is the only possible way in which to acquire the tricks so that at last they can be employed instantly and with all desired effec. tiveness. The student should begin by performing any one feat very slowly, and, while increase of speed is absolutely necessary, this increase should be very gradual, effort being concentrated on the knack of striking or fend. ing always with precision, to which even speed should be secondary for a long time—or until precision has become so much a matter of habit that speed will develop easily from it.

Practise at all odd times. When there are not more than two or three minutes of leisure, even, practise one of the feats and get a notch further ahead in its performance. Never get *out* of practise. *Jiu-jitsu* is not of so much use to the "rusty" adept. A Japanese teacher.

when he has no pupil on hand to instruct, will practise with any friend who may drop into the gymnasium. If there be no one present but himself, the teacher will take up something that he can do by himself.

One day, some years ago, the author stood chatting with a Japanese teacher of the art. Without warning the little brown man suddenly fell forward, his body as straight and rigid as a log. He fell squarely on his face, not putting out either hand to save himself. In a twinkling he was on his feet again.

"That is a good thing to be able to do," explained the teacher. "I was alone this morning, so I practised it by myself. And here is something else that it is worth while to know how to do."

With the same suddenness he fell over backward, his body as rigidly straight as before. And it seemed as if he had no more than touched the floor when he was on his feet once more.

All of the edge-of-the-hand blows seem so simple as to require but little practice. The reader who so concludes will make a huge mistake. These blows are so useful in a variety of cases that they should be practised with assiduity. It must be borne in mind that the boxer can strike rapidly. The *jiu-jitsian* must be able to use the edge of his hand with even greater speed.

The boxer must always bend—"flex"—and then extend his arm before he can deliver a telling blow. The *jiu-jitsian* will find that at times he has the great advantage of being able to use the edge-of-the-hand blow without bending his arm at all, and thus saving precious time in an encounter. If the hand, for instance, is hanging a little in front of the body, it can be made, by a single movement, to fly up and register a forcible blow against the adversary's jugular. A little experimenting will show the student a number of positions in which other edge-of-the-hand blows can be struck with a single movement of the arm — one upward, downward, or sideways. Never flex the arm when time can be saved by striking out without bending the arm.

The arm-hook is by no means unfamiliar to boxers, by whom it is regarded as a foul that is never to be employed except in rough-and-tumble. But photograph No. 14 shows how it is employed in *jiu-jitsu*. Here the man on the defensive has swung his right arm over the boxer's left in such fashion that a "hook" is made at the elbows. In the same moment the man on the defensive has swung his body around to the side in order to make the hook more effective, and he holds his left hand in readiness to strike an edge blow against the boxer's right wrist. As soon as the boxer's right comes the man on the defensive is ready to meet and stop it.

But the man on the defensive has also put himself in a first-rate position for assuming the offensive and putting an end to the fight. A single movement of the arm will enable him to dart his left hand upward from the boxer's right wrist and to deliver a finger-tip jab in the solar plexus or in the abdomen. The student will do well to note in how many other cases he is thus able to turn at once from the defensive to the aggressive and put an end to further attack by his opponent.

Photograph No. 15 depicts another style of

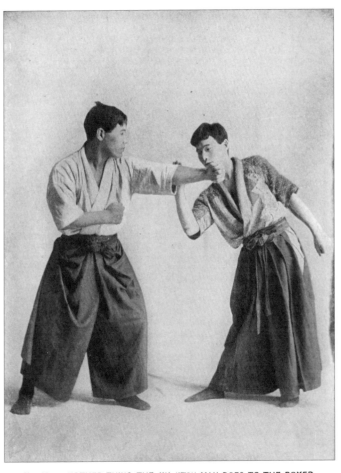

No. 16. ANOTHER THING THE JIU-JITSU MAN DOES TO THE BOXER.

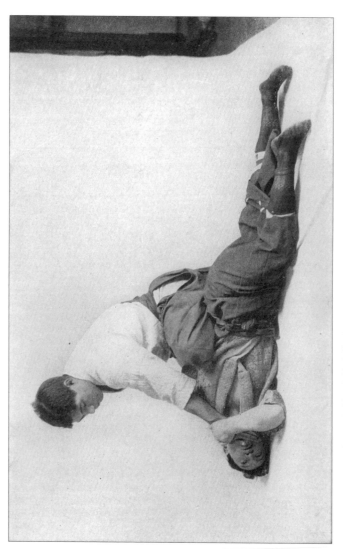

No. 17. THE CONVINCING FINISH OF DEFENSE SHOWN IN PRECEDING ILLUSTRATION.

defence against the boxer.   Here the *jiu-jitsian*
has struck up the boxer's left with the edge of
his own left hand, at the same instant ducking,
running in under the arm, and employing his
right hand in a vigorous edge-of-the-hand blow
over the boxer's left kidney.   This blow, when
well delivered, separates the boxer from any
desire to continue hostilities.

It is to be noted here that the *jiu-jitsian*
must accomplish the kidney blow with great
speed and enough force.   Otherwise the boxer
will have an opportunity of registering a dupli-
cate blow on the left kidney of his opponent.
It will be seen how easy it would be for the
boxer, if quick enough, and if dealing with a
slow adversary, to swing around and inflict his
own kidney blow.

When one is ducking under the boxer's arm
and striking the kidney blow it will easily occur
how simple it would be to strike, instead, at
the base of the spine.   But this latter is a
blow that should never be employed with the
edge of the hand.   It is decidedly too dangerous.   The base-of-the-spine blow, delivered at
a certain angle, and at a certain point of im-

pact, would probably result in leaving the combatant so struck bed-ridden for life.   In general it must be insisted that there is altogether too much danger in attacking the lower end of the spine with such a blow.

A considerable variety of blows in the abdomen, at the sides, and over the kidneys can be studied out by the industrious.   A general hint will be enough.   Any position that leaves a combatant's hand or elbow between the opponent's arm and body gives a valuable opportunity.   The fingers, the edge of the hand, or the point of the elbow may be used for swift attack against the soft parts.   The elbow, when in position, may be used effectively for a blow in the adversary's short ribs.

Nor must the use of the knee be forgotten when at close quarters.   A jab with the point of the knee may be employed against the abdomen or side when both hands are busy.   If one is behind his adversary he is often able to "butt" the point of one of his knees in over the kidney.   A kidney blow delivered with any force at all is one that discourages further fighting.

If one of the contestants is quick enough to
see and stop a rising knee from striking him, a
blow with the edge of the hand just above the
knee will be found very useful in forcing that
leg to straighten out again.

It is time, now, for the student who has
gone faithfully thus far to begin to study
out problems for himself.   He should, in
any given position of encounter, learn by
experiment how many of the holds and
blows he has so far learned may be applied
with effect, and which feats give better results than others.

It frequently happens that two antagonists
are practically locked—that is, assailant and
victim each has both arms employed, and for
either to let go would seem to expose him to
defeat.   In this position figure out all possible
ways of letting one hand go in order to make
an attack to advantage.   Or, if it is necessary
that both hands remain engaged where they
are, see whether a jab can be given with either
elbow.   Sometimes it will be found that the
point of the knee is the only weapon that can
be employed with safety against a vigilant

opponent. Whatever the strong factor is in the situation, find it and employ it at once—before the other man can find some disconcerting possibility.

CHAPTER VIII

ON THE GRADUAL ACQUIREMENT OF SPEED—
THE NEED OF WORKING, NOW, WITH AN
EXPERIENCED BOXER—TAKING A CLUB
AWAY FROM AN OPPONENT — AGILITY
GAINED BY THIS WORK—SIDE-STEPPING
AS SECOND NATURE

IT is time, right here, to call an earnest halt
against the natural impulse of the student
to try to learn, in one or two bouts of practice,
all of the principal feats that are employed in
stopping the boxer. In instructing his friends
the author has discovered the difficulty of convincing a student that a new feat, once men-
tally grasped, is by no means *mastered*.

If the reader has the patience and perse-
verance that he should bring to this work I will
offer him a suggestion that is of great value.
Do not attempt to learn more than one trick
at a time; do not be in haste to go to another.
Several bouts of practice should be devoted to

the repeated—even if monotonous—rehearsal of the feat that is under consideration. *Jiu-jitsu* tricks, in order to be of real value to their possessor, must become in their execution as second nature. The student who departs from this rule, and who tries to make haste, will be sorry for it later on.

It has been stated already that the first *desideratum* is to be able to execute a feat with unvarying precision. Make sure that you can always perform the feat in exactly the same way. Precision counts for nearly everything in the effect that is to be produced on the opponent.

Pay so much attention to precision as not to be in haste to get up speed. When precision has become second nature, then speed will follow quickly. Do not try for speed until it is unnecessary any longer to pay particular attention to the matter of precision.

At this point there is another mistake of which most students are naturally guilty, and it is one that should be rigorously avoided. When working, at last, for speed, do not feel that, for the time being, the matter of precision

may be overlooked in favour of rapidity of execution. *Never, even temporarily, slight precision
for the sake of speed.* Consider the gaining of
speed as a matter of no importance when it is
acquired at the least expense in the way of precision. After all, patience and the willingness
to progress only as rapidly as is consistent with
thorough work are the most valuable traits for
the student to possess at this point in his
training.

After the work of picking up speed, as an
addition only to precision, has been gotten
fairly under way, it is much better for the student if he can practise with a man well versed
in boxing. The boxer, when he has seen the
jiu-jitsu method of stopping him, will be able
to suggest many other ways in which he might
have an opportunity of downing the *jiu-jitsian.*
And thus, by practice and study against the
traps of the boxer, the student is able to teach
himself much.

Bear in mind always that speed has not been
developed to perfection until the *jiu-jitsian* is
able to stop a rapid and skilled boxer. It is
possible for any agile student to reach this

stage of development, for the feats that are employed against the boxer can all be used with greater swiftness than is possible in delivering boxing blows. Hence the student will know when he has gained the right amount of speed with a given feat; it is when he is able to move quickly enough to prevent the boxer from defeating him.

And the student should constantly encourage his boxing companion to suggest all possible ways of delivering the blow so that *jiu-jitsu* might not stop it. This affords rugged and varied drill for the novice in *jiu-jitsu*.

Of course agility is one of the main factors in gaining speed, although it is not the only requisite. Quick vision, intelligence, and a very considerable degree of automatism are also needed. For making agility there is no better exercise than practising the feat of taking away a club from an opponent who makes an attack with that weapon. Nor is it at all difficult to learn how to get the club every time.

In the beginning have your opponent stand facing you with the bludgeon in his right hand.

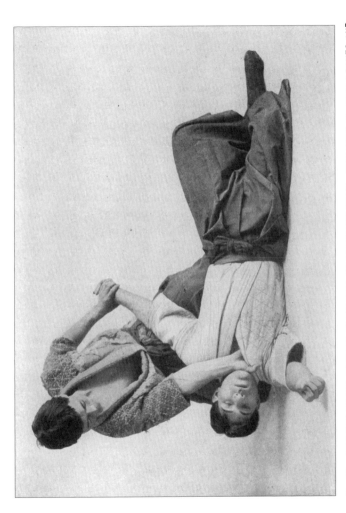

No. 18.   ANOTHER USEFUL METHOD OF HOLDING AN OPPONENT DOWN—EMPLOYED AGAINST A BOXER AND IN WRESTLING.

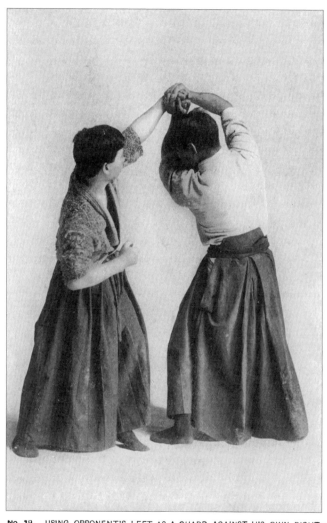

No. 19. USING OPPONENT'S LEFT AS A GUARD AGAINST HIS OWN RIGHT—
THIS FEAT ENDS IN A THROW.

Have him raise this weapon and bring it down across the top of your head — or, at least, *attempt* so to strike you. Of course, at the outset, the assailant does not attempt to strike quickly, increasing the rapidity of the blow only with the *jiu-jitsian's* acquirement of speed in stopping him.

The student's defence consists in throwing up his left hand and seizing the wrist of the hand that holds the club. The wrist is seized from underneath. At the moment of taking this hold the student grabs the club with his right hand. The assailant's hand is held, just as it is caught, with the thumb side of the hand up. With his right hand the man on the defensive twists the club over and downward, back of the hand, at the same time retaining a strong, vise-like hold on the wrist. The twist on the club forces it out of the hand of the assailant. Your true *jiu-jitsian*, on securing the club, throws it away and carries on the battle with Nature's weapons.

By degrees the student becomes so well assured of his ability to catch and to hold the assailant's right wrist that the attacking man

can at last deliver the blow with all the speed
of which he is capable. And the man on the
defensive catches the wrist and twists away the
club so quickly that the assailant is deprived of
his weapon before he has had time to realise it.

When the ability to take the club away at
lightning-like speed has been fully acquired,
the student should vary his practice by asking
the adversary to strike at any part of the body,
and from any direction. It does not require
much added practice to render the student
practically proof against assault with a club.
But it must be borne in mind at all times that
the assailant's hand must be so caught as to
leave the thumb side of the hand up; and that
the club must be twisted downward over the
back of the hand.

Another feat that makes for agility, and one
that saves the student the discomfort of many
a blow received, is that of side-stepping.
Practise this, at first, by letting your adversary
strike out at you without much speed. Suppose he strikes for your face, or your chin,
with his left hand? Take one quick step to
your own left—to the right of *his* body. His

blow will pass harmlessly by you.   Keep at
this side-stepping patiently until you execute
it as a matter of second nature.

Then ask your boxing friend to increase the
speed of his blow gradually, and keep at it
until you are able to side-step out of the way
of the swiftest blow that he can send out.   Be
satisfied, in the end, with nothing less than the
speed that enables you to step easily away
from his swiftest blow.   And this speed in
side-stepping can be acquired without fail if
the practice is patient enough, and if the *jiu-
jitsian* is ever keenly alert.

But in side-stepping out of the way of the
boxer's left-hander always bear in mind that
he has a chance to follow up and register with
a right-hander.   In side-stepping have your
own left hand in readiness to stop his right by
a sharp edge-of-the-hand blow across his right
fore-arm.

In side-stepping out of harm's way there is
an opportunity, at the same time, to deprive
the boxer of any further interest in the contest.   While stepping, let your right hand go
up with a rapid sweep, the little-finger edge

striking him fully and forcibly across the right jugular. If this blow lands with force and sharpness enough any man other than a Hercules will go to the floor. Even when lightly delivered this blow makes the recipient feel uncomfortable.

But there is still another trick to side-stepping. Follow up the first step with a quick second step in the same direction. Thus, if anything happens that prevents your blow from landing on your opponent's neck, the second side-step carries you out of the reach of any blow he may send suddenly after you.

Pay great attention at all times to practice in this side-stepping. It offers the most effective means, when thoroughly mastered, of getting out of harm's way, or, at the worst, of minimising the effect of any blow that the boxer may succeed in landing. *Jiu-jitsu*, without swift and effective side-stepping, is not *jiu-jitsu* at all.

CHAPTER IX

EXPONENTS of the Ten-jin school of *jiu-jitsu* have developed in all its possible
perfection a style of stopping the boxer's blow
that cannot be surpassed for neatness of execution, effectiveness, and swiftness. It is a
feat that applies only to stopping a left-hand
blow by the boxer.

This trick of defence may be taken up in
three stages, and I shall describe each stage by
itself. After the student has mastered all three
of the stages he can combine them all in rapid
succession, with the result that he is able to
stop the blow and to have his opponent on the

floor, helpless, but not in any way disabled.
The entire length of time employed in this feat
should not exceed four or five seconds.

Just as the boxer launches his left fist
"duck" quickly to his left, taking your own
head and upper trunk out of danger. At the
same time strike the outer bend of his left
elbow with the open palm of the right hand.
The manner of dodging and of striking the
assailant's elbow is shown clearly in photograph No. 16.

Always strike the adversary's elbow with a
smart, forceful blow. The effect will be to
send him spinning around to his own right.
The very momentum that the boxer gives himself in striking forward will aid in swinging him
around.

This ward-off at the elbow must be practised
over and over again. It is easy to give this
fend-off with fair speed, but this will not meet
the demands of actual combat. *Extreme* speed
must be developed, and this is why the trick
must be practised for a long time, and with
very patient attention to gaining speed.

Both the dodging and the striking of the

elbow are to be persisted in until nothing is left
to be desired in the performance.   And try to
swing the assailant farther and farther around.

In actual combat the effect of this first stage
of the trick is amusing on the assailant who
knows nothing of *jiu-jitsu*, and who is not prepared to receive such a fend-off.   When he
finds that he cannot land his blow, and that he
is sent spinning around as often as he tries it,
he loses confidence in himself.   He realises
that he is at the mercy of his opponent.

Now comes the second stage of the trick, the
throw.   This must be begun the instant that
the adversary has been fended off and sent
spinning around to his right.   Clap your right
hand smartly over his right kidney.   At the
same time your left arm goes up under his extended left.   Your left hand must rest on his
right shoulder, taking a quick grip there, and
the length of your left arm, of course, is across
his chest.

Just the instant that this hold has been obtained—and it must be while your assailant is
still spinning to his right—force him over backward to the ground.   It will not be at all diffi-

cult, for his own momentum in his forced swing around will help carry him as you wish him to go. And thus the second stage of the trick ends with the assailant lying on the ground.

Now, this second part of the feat is to be acquired very painstakingly. Practise over and over again the getting of the hold with each hand just as it has been described. Remember, too, that the right hand on the adversary's kidney should press him forward, while the left arm across his chest should force him over backward. And be sure that the left hand always grips at the right shoulder of your antagonist. Make sure, also, that you strike him so smartly over the kidney as to cause pain and weakness there. Having gotten hold just right with each of your hands, the matter of throwing does not require such close attention. The antagonist is thrown to the ground with no trouble whatever if the holds are taken properly and if the backward pressure is used without an instant's delay.

The thrown opponent will land either on his back, or on his right side. This depends much upon the way the pressure against him is

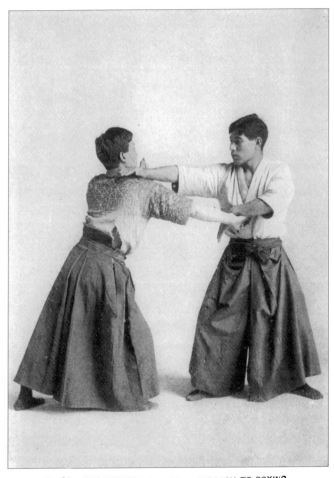

No. 20.   THE NEAREST JIU-JITSU APPROACH TO BOXING.

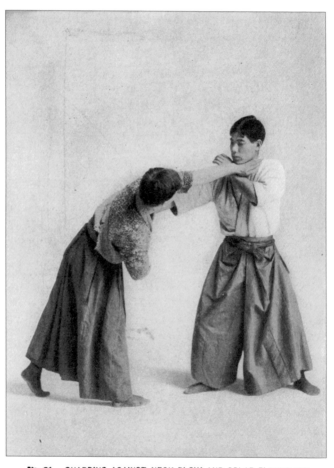

No. 21. GUARDING AGAINST NECK BLOW AND SOLAR-PLEXUS JAB.

applied. It depends to some extent, also, on the nature of the resistance that he makes against being thrown.

In photograph No. 17 the defeated man is shown lying on his right side. His head is held firmly to the ground by his victorious antagonist's left hand. The victor's left knee has been jabbed into the victim's short ribs as the victor fell a-top of him. This has driven the breath out of the defeated man. But the victor does not stop here, for the prostrate man will have his breath soon, and will be able to renew the contest. It is necessary, therefore, to reduce the victim to complete submission.

The victor's right hand has clutched the victim's left wrist. The captured left arm is held across the victor's right knee, which is under the upper half of the captured arm. The inside of the victim's wrist is upward, and the victor is pressing the wrist down forcibly. The effect of this is to make the captured arm bend over the victor's knee, and to bend in just the opposite way from that which Nature intended. If this pressure be given hard enough the effect will be to break the bone of the left upper arm. But, instead, the victor contents himself with straining the captured arm with somewhat rapidly increasing severity until the pain in that arm becomes so intense that the defeated man signifies his complete surrender.

Here is the trick, now, in its three stages, and the whole combination, from the first "duck" to the straining of the defeated man's left arm, should be performed in about four or five seconds. It should be practised and practised until this speed has been reached, for this feat offers the best all-around defence against the boxer that is known to the *jiu-jitsian*.

When the man who is thrown lands on his back, the left knee of the victor is planted at the left edge of the abdomen. It is important for the victor to remember to employ his left hand in forcing the head of his fallen antagonist to the floor, as otherwise the latter will be able to secure some purchase for rising, or will be able to lift his head sufficiently to inflict, possibly, a disconcerting bite—for biting is employed, as a last resort, in *jiu-jitsu*, as in all other styles of fighting the world over.

It is worth while to call attention again to

the theory of breaking the arm.   The Japanese
call it "breaking," even when nothing more
than straining the arm is attempted.   The inside of the wrist *must* be upward, and the
pressure against the upper bone of the arm
applied in the opposite direction to that in
which the arm was made by Nature to bend.
This would bring the knee under the back of
the upper arm.

With one experiment it will be seen that if
the straining of the arm is applied with the inside of the wrist downward the only effect will
be to bend the arm in the natural way and the
victim will not be hurt thereby.

A very clear idea of how the arm is strained
or broken is afforded by photograph No. 18.
This illustrates, also, a hold that is employed
with advantage when an opponent has been
thrown after either boxing or wrestling.

The victor has his right arm under the victim's left.   The victor's right hand clutches at
the shirt (or vest or coat) of the fallen man,
and in such manner that the knuckles of the
hand press severely against the ribs close to
the right shoulder.

Careful study of the illustration will show that the victim's captured left arm is held over the straight, rigid right arm of the victor, and that it is the back of the victim's left arm that is pressed against the other's arm. Now, by applying downward pressure at the captured left wrist the victor is able to cause a great deal of pain, and, if he makes the downward pressure a vicious one, the assailant is able to break his opponent's arm above the elbow.

Note that the fulcrum applied by the assailant to the back of the victim's arm, whether that fulcrum be an arm or a knee, is always applied well above the elbow. A little experimenting with this straining of the arm will show why this should be so.

More is to be said, later on, about this work of straining a victim's arm, or breaking it if need be, and in the meantime the student is advised to give some study to the positions of the contestants as shown in photographs Nos. 23 to 25, in which other feats are shown where the same principle of attack or defence is employed.

CHAPTER X

THERE is something well-nigh humorous
in the style of combat that is shown in
photograph No. 19. It is worthy of the best
traditions of Oriental subtlety and ingenuity
that the boxer should be forced to defeat
himself.

During the study of this text and the first
practising of the feat it will be well to make
frequent reference to the illustration. The
pose is so perfect that it offers answers to
many of the questions that the student will ask
of himself.

In this particular bit of work a well-trained
eye and vimful agility are all-important. The

trick is worthless as a means of actual defence
until all the requirements of speed have been
brought out by frequent and all but unremitting practice.

The feat begins with a defence against the
boxer's left-hand blow. The man on the defensive must shoot both of his hands forward
and upward at the coming left hand of the opponent. The hands of the man on the defensive are well together, very much in the form
of a "V," although the heels of the hands do
not quite touch. It is this "V" that is shot
up to catch and encircle the boxer's fist—*not
his wrist !* At the instant that the assailant's
fist is caught in this "V" the man on the defensive wraps his fingers around the captured
fist.

Reference to the photograph will show just
how this encircling of the attacking fist is accomplished. One point the illustration does
not show exactly, and no amount of author's
text can explain it fully; and that is just how
to hold the attacking fist so that its owner
cannot wrench it free. But such a hold can
be taken and the student, by a little patient

experimenting, can learn just how to get this hold of the fist, and—better still—how to retain it. All through the work with this trick it must be remembered that the man on the defensive has the resources of *two hands* to employ against the power of *one fist*.

Now, the man who has captured his adversary's fist must be prepared to move that fist wherever he wants it to go in front or at the side of the owner's body. It may seem that the owner of the captured fist can block this movement by exerting the muscles of his left arm to their utmost, but again it is to be pointed out that the man on the defensive has all the strength of two arms with which to oppose whatever strength his opponent can put into one arm.

"But when the fellow's left fist is caught what will he do with that idle right fist?" is a question that the reader will be sure to ask.

The answer is a simple one: "The fellow will do nothing of any importance with his idle right fist."

It is here that the essence of the trick comes in. Let the man strike out with his right fist.

The man on the defensive brings that captured
fist and its arm swiftly down, crossing the fore-
arm of that captured fist over the fore-arm of
the opponent's assailing right. It is a complete block, stopping the boxer's blow. And
the same manœuvre will stop any blow that
the boxer can try to deliver with his right.
Wherever the right fist tries to land it is
blocked by contact with the fore-arm behind
the captured fist. It is impossible to make
any striking blow with the right that cannot be
stopped by swift contact with the captured
left.

Always the man on the defensive forces, up
or down, the boxer's left arm so that it is made
to cross the boxer's right, the point of contact
being in the fore-arms of the boxer. There is
no escape for the boxer, and he is made to
submit to the humiliation of practically warding off his own blows.

And not only are the blows stopped, but
there is actual mischief in this style of defence,
for the boxer's fore-arms are brought together
so sharply that each concussion causes pain,
and three or four sharp impacts leave the

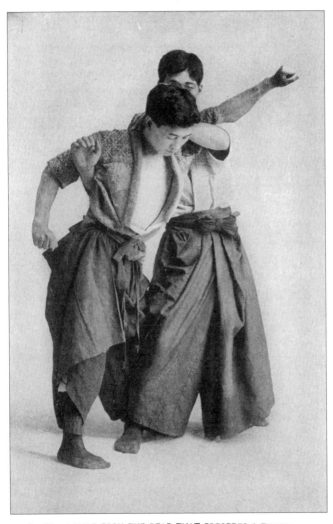

No. 22.   A HOLD FROM THE REAR **THAT** PRECEDES A **T**HROW.

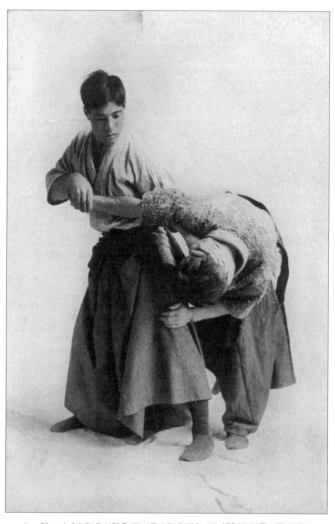

No. 23   A SIMPLE HOLD THAT RENDERS AN ASSAILANT HELPLESS.

boxer very sick of this style of defeat. His arms are badly lamed, and he is not likely to care for any more boxing for a few hours.

But there is still more mischief in this defence, for, at any time, at the pleasure of the man on the defensive, he can throw his adversary and thus put an end to tactics that have furnished sport but for one. And the throw is accomplished very easily. Bring the boxer's left arm down to ward off a blow from his right. At the instant of impact wrench that captured left arm up smartly so that the fist is brought higher than the boxer's head. Do not hold it there, but carry on the movement so that the left arm of the boxer is forced far out to his left side and down with a wrench. At the same time something of a twist is given to the wrist behind the captured fist, and the whole movement wrenches the boxer off his balance and sends him to the ground. Once he is there, he may be left to regain his footing, or he may be effectually subdued by any of the tricks already described that have that end in view.

This is the whole combination of the clever

movement—catching the fist as it is struck out, forcing the arm down to parry a blow by the right hand, and then instantly forcing the captured fist up, over to the left, way out at the side and down toward the ground, throwing the boxer. From the instant that the fist is captured to the instant when the boxer is down should not take up more than three seconds. This speed is easily acquired with practice.

The first thing to learn to do well is to catch the boxer's left fist. At first the practice should not go beyond this point. Using the ward-off against the boxer's right is a matter so simple as to require but a small amount of practice, and the same may be said of the arm-wrench that accomplishes the throw. So that the only points in this work calling for assiduous practice are the catching of the fist and mastering the way of holding it so that the boxer cannot yank his fist free.

Boxing is so natural a method of personal combat that it is not to be supposed that the ancient Japanese never thought of employing it. But the Japanese has improved upon our method of striking with the clenched fist. He found out, some twenty-five hundred years ago, that far more damaging blows may be struck with the sharp, hardened edge of the hand than are possible with the blunt, wide-surfaced fist.

And this work with the edge of the hand is the nearest approach to boxing that *jiu-jitsu* offers. The movements of the arms are very similar to those of the boxer, but the blows with the edge of the hand are sharp and sting-ing, and often break one of the adversary's bones. The work shown in photograph No. 20 gives an excellent idea of this work. Each contestant has tried to land an edge-of-the-hand blow on his adversary's neck or throat, and each has parried with the edge of the hand on guard. Neither man has succeeded in registering, and both are open for the next move of attack or of defence.

In photograph No. 21, one man is shown striking for the side of the neck, while the other endeavours to land a finger-tip jab in the solar plexus. Both attacks are defeated by an edge-of-the-hand guard. In this work, as in boxing, feinting is resorted to as a means of landing a blow, but *jiu-jitsians* are so agile and so quick of eye that a feinted jab or blow is followed rarely by one that registers. As a rule, when this hand-work imitation of boxing is attempted it is carried on merely as a sort of "sparring for wind," each antagonist being keenly on the alert for an opening that shall make it possible to secure one of the holds that are so much more effective.

Always in the clinch that follows this *ad-interim* sparring the *jiu-jitsian* tries for an opportunity to bring the edge of his hand sharply against the opponent's collar-bone, causing great pain there, or even fracturing the bone.

In clinches, and, in fact, in any position where one of the men has the point of his elbow close to the ribs, or to the soft parts of the trunk, he gives a sharp jab with the elbow, the blow having much the same effect that would result from the blow of the boxer's fist.

A blow that is peculiarly annoying to the opponent is one that is struck slantingly across the forehead with the edge of the hand. If this blow be landed three or four times during a bout of combat, the man who is punished will be certain of a spell of headache. There is no actual danger from this blow if it is struck temperately, but of course it becomes highly dangerous when struck with great force.

Edge-of-the-hand blows may be practised lightly across the temples, and just over the ears. In fact these blows should be frequently employed — lightly — in practice bouts. In actual combat, however, these two blows should never be brought into use unless it is absolutely necessary, in a position of great danger, to employ them, for both are more than ordinarily dangerous.

The true jiu-jitsian is never a bully. He never strikes a dangerous blow with anything like full force unless he believes himself to be justified by extreme necessity. The aim is not to disable needlessly, but to convince an adversary of the folly of carrying the fight further. And it is the height of the chivalry of jiu-jitsu to end the fight the instant that the defeated combatant betrays the fact that he has had punishment enough.

Extreme consideration for the physical pains

and the mental feelings of an enemy should lie at the foundation of *jiu-jitsu*.   In feudal Japan the law dealt severely with an adept who used his knowledge of the art for bullying or other improper purposes.

CHAPTER XI

TWO SAFE, CERTAIN, AND EASY HOLDS FOR
REDUCING AN OPPONENT—STRAINING AN
ADVERSARY'S ARM OVER THE SHOULDER
—HOW THE VICTORY MAY BE FOLLOWED
UP WITH A THROW IN EITHER OF THE
THREE CASES

WRESTLERS have a hold known as the
"Nelson." The ancient originators
of *jiu-jitsu* devised a hold that is somewhat
similar, and the essential principle of the
Japanese style of hold is shown clearly in
photograph No. 22.

As in American or English wrestling, the
assailant secures the hold from behind. The
assailant's left arm is thrown under the victim's
left arm, forcing that latter member up, and
the assailant's hand is pressed against the back
of the victim's neck, the fingers gripping at
the right. At the same time the assailant's
right hand and fore-arm are thrust under the

victim's right shoulder and the back of the hand is held pressing against the shoulder. No further description of the hold will be needed, the illustration showing just how it is taken.

This feat may be used as a hold pure and simple, for the purposes of keeping the victim helpless. In the case that the assailant is standing behind the victim, the latter has a slight means of defence and counter by kicking the aggressor's shins with the back of one heel. But if the assailant is on the alert for this demonstration he can squelch it by stepping nimbly back and dragging his victim backward to the ground.

When this trick is used as a hold the victim's head is forced forward and down, while the assailant's right hand drags the victim's right shoulder backward. The victim is thus helpless at his opponent's pleasure, unless the victim resorts to the back-heel kick, and it has been explained how this is met by the aggressor. Or, the victim may try to bend far forward so as to lift the assailant from his feet, but in this case the assailant can rapidly shift his hold to

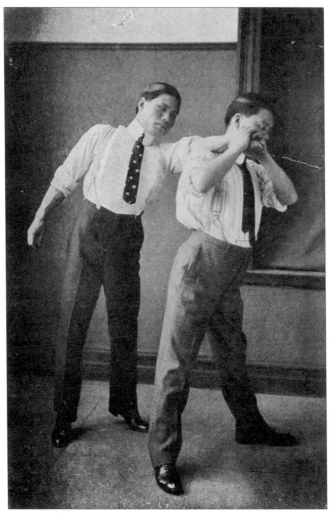

No. 24.   STRAINING A FOREARM OVER THE SHOULDER.

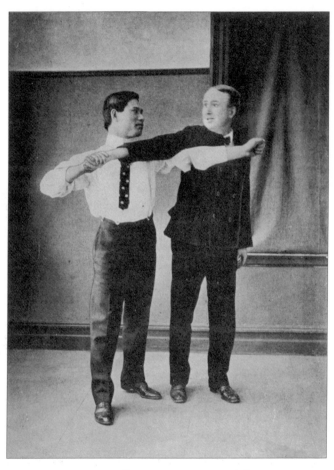

No. 25. "THE DEVIL'S HAND-SHAKE."

one with both hands at the front of the victim's throat, and the aggressor is then in a position to choke his victim and drag him over backward.

But when it is intended, from the outset, to throw the victim, the assailant, at the moment of taking the hold, advances his right leg in front of the victim's left. The head is forced forward and down, and the victim's right shoulder is wrenched violently upward. With this combination it is a matter of ease to throw the victim over the leg.

A hold that may be retained at the position of seizing, or that may be carried on to a throw, is all but explained by a glance at photograph No. 23. In this feat the assailant, with his right hand, seizes the victim's right wrist. At the same time the assailant's left arm is forced under the victim's right arm. This combination of attack makes it possible to throw up the victim's right arm. The inner, or palm side of the victim's wrist is held upward. The assailant's left hand is pressed squarely over the back of the victim's head, and the head is forced down to the ground.

Now, note the position of the victim's captured right arm. The inside of the wrist of that arm being held up, and the hand being forced downward, it follows that the victim's right arm is being made to bend the "wrong way." Thus the captured arm will be severely strained; it may even be broken if the pressure is ugly enough. It is important for the assailant always to remember to hold the captured right arm of his opponent in the way indicated, and to apply the straining pressure with sufficient force to reduce the victim to surrender. As to the throw, it may be accomplished by forcing the victim's head down and down until he collapses on the floor—all the while applying the strain to his captured right arm. The chances are that before the victim is forced to the ground he will call out his surrender, but much depends upon the force with which his right arm is strained—and it cannot be strained at all unless the assailant has paid attention to the method of doing it. In throwing, if desired, the assailant may give a trip over his own left leg.

This hold is so important in a variety of

conditions of combat that it should be practised
long and faithfully, until the student feels certain that he is able to perform it as well as he
could do even if he were to add much more
practice.   While the feat is of great value to
any one who may become involved in a personal
encounter, and who desires to end it quickly,
the attention of police officers is called to this
trick as an effective one in subduing a troublesome prisoner.   It is swifter and more effective
than clubbing—and decidedly more humane.
The victim, after he has been subdued, will
know better than to attempt further trouble
with a master of such tricks, and the prisoner
will not have been mangled or battered, but
will feel as comfortable as he did before this
assault was made upon him.

A plucky and reasonably muscular woman
would find this trick useful in taking care of an
intruder whom she found in her home during
the absence of her male protectors.   The intruder could be seized and held, without throwing, until help arrived, and sufficient straining
of the intruder's right arm would cause him
to hope as ardently as would the woman for

the speedy arrival of the help summoned by
screams.

In the practice of this trick care must be
taken to avoid fumbling. The difficulty that
the novice experiences is in getting his left
arm surely and swiftly under the victim's
right. If the victim's opposition be quick and
determined the neophyte in *jiu-jitsu* will find
it hard to get his left arm under and the hand
securely fixed against the back of the victim's
head. Yet this must be done surely and well,
since the left hand not only presses the victim's
head down, but also gives the leverage that results in the successful straining of the victim's
right arm. Practice, therefore, should be per-
sistent until the new *jiu-jitsian* is able to secure
the hold without the suspicion of a fumble.

As to the victim's counter, the only one that
is possible, once the hold has been securely
taken, is to grip at the muscles of the aggressor's left leg and to try to inflict pain there.
If this is attempted the assailant should increase the straining pressure on his adversary's
right arm and make the throw at once.

In proper sequence comes the feat of straining an adversary's arm over the shoulder. This can be applied in a variety of cases, and if used severely enough it is a means of promptly ending an encounter. The position is depicted in photograph No. 24.

The attack may be made under any one of a variety of circumstances. Whenever the opponent's arm is extended toward you seize his wrist firmly with both hands, forcing the inside of his wrist upward, and holding it so. At the instant of so seizing the wrist and turning it, swing swiftly around so as to present your back to the opponent. Swing your shoulder under the upper half of his captured arm, and bear down heavily at the wrist. Thus his arm is forced to bend the "wrong way," and the enormous leverage possessed by the aggressor will enable the latter to inflict pain to any degree up to the unbearable. The victim can be forced to stand upon the tips of his toes.

If it is wished, a throw can be made. All the assailant has to do is to bend well over forward, and, with his pull on the victim's arm, to send the latter flying over his shoulder. But this style of throw may result in a broken arm for the victim, and for this reason the throw should never be employed except in a desperate case. But the throw may be *practised*, nevertheless, by bending forward and sending the victim part way over the shoulder, then straightening up again and permitting the victim to regain his feet.

Right here it is important to make one point clear to the student of *jiu-jitsu*. In pulling the victim's arm over the shoulder, make sure that you bring his left arm over your right shoulder, or his right arm over your left shoulder. Otherwise the trick is pretty certain to end in defeat for the aggressor. Suppose, for instance, that you blunderingly take the assailant's right arm over your right shoulder. Then he is in position to use his disengaged left hand in giving you a disastrous blow in the back or over the kidneys. If you take his left arm over your left shoulder the victim has an opportunity to use his right hand in a similar fashion.

Study the illustration once more, and it will be understood that by taking the captured left arm over your right shoulder, or the right arm over your left shoulder, the victim is deprived of his opportunity of countering. This point must always be remembered.

If an antagonist seizes the coat lapel this hold may be instantly taken. If he has seized your throat with one hand, or is reaching for it, the hold can be taken and the painful pressure applied before the adversary has time to realise what is about to happen. If an adversary pushes you away the hold comes into instant play. If he tries to drag you by the coat collar, bring his arm over your shoulder.

This trick can be employed, too, in connection with the trick of catching the boxer's fist that was described in the last chapter. If he strikes at you, the instant that you have imprisoned his fist, swing and bring his arm over your shoulder—always *remembering* that the inside of his wrist must be upward.

Now, it will happen often that at the moment of sending his hand your way the opponent will have the inside of his wrist downward. Study, therefore, the best method of seizing his wrist in order to have free play for turning the inside of his wrist upward. And, as the adversary will naturally try to keep his wrist from being twisted, a good deal of practice must be devoted to so turning his wrist that you can always have the opponent's wrist turned upward, and his arm over your shoulder, before he has had time to understand the nature of the trick that you intend to play upon him.

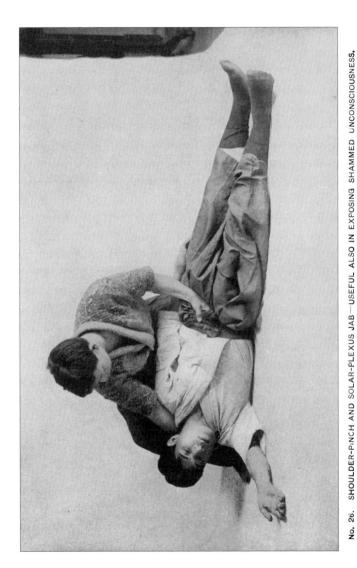

No. 26. SHOULDER-PINCH AND SOLAR-PLEXUS JAB—USEFUL ALSO IN EXPOSING SHAMMED UNCONSCIOUSNESS.

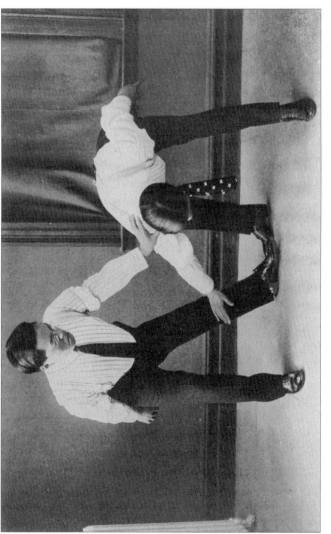

No 27. PREVENTING AN INJURY TO KNEE OR OTHER CONTIGUOUS PARTS.

CHAPTER XII

UNDER certain conditions nearly all of the tricks of *jiu-jitsu* have their humorous aspects. This is true especially when a trick is employed with just enough force so that the victim is not made to suffer any pain, but is made to realise how helpless he would be if the feat were employed against him in earnest. And there are some tricks that are more than ordinarily humorous.

One that is of great value for combat pur-poses, but which will afford a good deal of amusement is that of stopping any one in his walk by the use only of the forefinger. If you meet a friend who is walking in the direction opposite to that which you are following, stop just as you reach him. Stand at his side and extend an arm, holding the forefinger under his nose and across his upper lip. If you stand still, and hold the finger in that position, he will find it impossible to walk by you. Of course he is able to move his head to one side and resume his walk, but as long as the forefinger is under his nose he cannot get by. There is no trick about this. It is simply the consequence of a natural law. But it will afford a good deal of amusement, for your friend will be unable to understand why there is not more power in his whole body than in your forefinger.

Once in a great while you will encounter a man so powerful that he will be able slowly to get by you. Now, the back of your hand is up. Turn the back of the hand over toward his face, "grinding" the forefinger under his nose, and this added power will be enough to stop the progress of the strongest man.

It would seem impossible to hurt a policeman severely with his own club, and that without drawing the club from his belt. Yet it is a very simple and effective trick, and is easily performed. A good deal of amusement can be had when the trick is played on a friendly policeman, although it might be bad judgment to try it upon an officer who had a strong sense of dignity coupled with little appreciation of humour.

Step behind the policeman when his club is hanging in its accustomed loop at the left side of his belt. Seize his left wrist with your left hand, and hold that wrist firmly, at the same time raising the arm sideways a little. Seize the lower end of his club with your right hand, and pull it back, upward and over, making the club stand nearly upside down in the loop. The shaft of the club is to be pressed hard against the back of his left arm at a point just above the elbow. The inside of his captured wrist is toward the front.

Now, with your left hand pull his wrist backward, at the same time pressing forward against the back of his upper arm with the club. This combined pressure makes his arm bend the "wrong way." If you were to pull backward severely enough at his wrist, and press forward hard enough with the club, probably you would break his arm.

But it is not necessary to do this. As soon as the policeman realises how ruthlessly he is held he will give in good naturedly if he understands that it is all a joke. Try the trick, and you will soon see why he cannot do anything with his right hand in the way of swinging around upon you with a blow. If he tries to he will merely increase the amount of pain in his captured and oppressed left arm.

By pushing slowly forward with the inverted club, and all the while pulling back on his wrist, it will be possible to make the officer bend forward to the ground, and it is possible, even, to throw him directly in this fashion. Even if there be any difficulty in making him lie down, a trip with your right foot against his left will send him prostrate. Nor is the trick at an end as a piece of humour when you have thrown your good-natured policeman. There is one bit more of fun in store for you and for the policeman—provided his sense of the ridiculous has not been overtaxed.   In throwing hold the club so that the head of it will be twisted into a position in front of his abdomen, and he falls with his abdomen pressing against the head of the club.

His left arm is on the ground; the head of the club is under his abdomen, and the shaft passes over his arm; your right hand is near the lower end of the club.   The policeman's arm will serve as a fulcrum, his club as a lever, your right arm as the power, and his unfortunate abdomen as the weight.   Press down on the bottom of the club, and the head of the club is bound to rise, pressing roughly against his abdomen.   His arm as well as his abdomen will suffer.

If the directions are carefully followed, and the trick be practised thoroughly, a guarantee goes with the performance of the feat.   The same piece of mischief may be played on a military officer who is wearing his sword at his side.   Practise the trick by tying a girdle around a friend's waist and passing a stout stick through the girdle.   Read this text over carefully, practising the trick step by step until you have it mastered, and bearing in mind, always, that the victim's wrist must be kept to the front so that the arm will be made to bend "the wrong way."

As it is quite within the bounds of possibility that a law-breaker might attempt this trick in earnest against a policeman, it is only fair to the blue-coat to advise him as to the counter that must be employed. The next paragraph, therefore, is addressed to the policeman.

Get a friend to seize your wrist and club and place you in the hold already described, omitting the throw. As soon as you feel yourself seized *bend slightly forward.* The forward bend should be just sufficient to enable you to carry out the further directions that are to be given. Still in bending position, twist your right leg and the right side of your trunk around in front of your assailant. Your right leg should be bent a little, and the front of the upper part of this leg should be slantingly across the front of the assailant's left leg just above his knee. Pass your right hand in front of the aggressor's right leg, and around in back of it just above the knee. The thumb side of this hand should be down, so that you are able to take a grip at the back of his leg, just above the knee, with the thumb pressing the back of the leg, and the fingers of the hand gripping the inside of his leg. It may be preferred to pass the hand around the inside of the leg and gripping at the back of the knee. Having obtained this position, rise with a jerking movement to an erect position, and follow this by bending over backward. Then the assailant who thought he had you will find himself thrown over backward.

And, as the policeman will find that there will be many abroad in the land who will try the assault upon him in a more or less humorous way, it behooves him to practise this effective counter most diligently.

It is best, too, that the policeman should acquire another trick that will make his work easier. Here is a feat that is valuable to all *jiu-jitsians*, and it will enable a policeman to force a troublesome prisoner into going along with him.

In *Japanese Physical Training* the author

has described the "come along." This trick is sometimes varied in the following manner:

With the left hand seize the intended victim's left wrist while standing at his left side and facing in the same direction that he is looking. Draw his left arm toward your own left side. At the same time throw your right arm over his right arm, and then under the upper half of his right arm. Rest your right hand on your abdomen. See to it that the inside of his left wrist, which you hold with your left hand, is up. Now, press downward against his left wrist, forcing his left arm to "bend the wrong way." Now, you can force the victim forward, and he will be glad enough to go where he is ordered to go. If he attempts to hang back, increase the pressure on, and the pain in, his left arm, and he will surrender. He cannot strike with his right hand, for you control his movements from his left side.

The same principle of causing pain by making the arm "bend the wrong way " is at the bottom of the bit of mischief known as "the devil's hand-shake." Photograph No. 25 makes the operation of the trick clear.

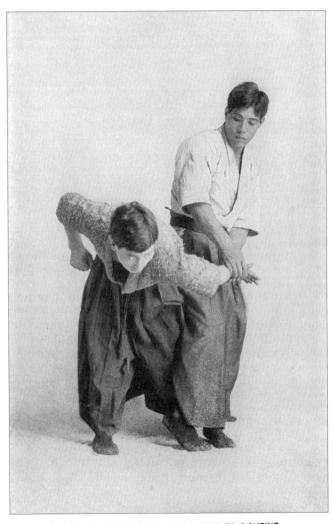

No. 28.   STRAINING AN ARM AS A STOP TO FIGHTING.

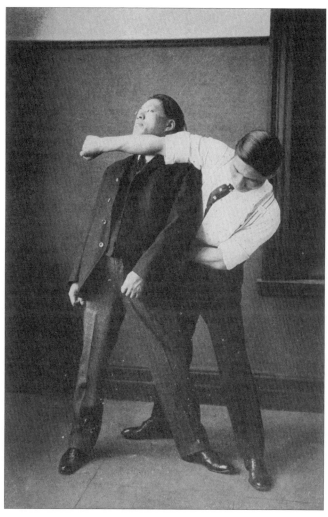

No. 29. A FEAT USED EITHER AS A HOLD OR FOR A THROW.

Approach the intended victim and take his right hand in your own as if about to shake hands with him. Throw his arm up, swing around at his side, and at the same time thrust your extended, rigid left arm under his captured right. Your left arm will assist in throwing his right arm up. See to it that the inside of his wrist is uppermost. The illustration will make this plain.

Now, bear down on his right hand while holding the victim's arm up with your own rigid left arm. There will be a quick shoot of pain through the victim's captured arm, and it is possible to apply the pressure so severely that he will rise on his toes. If you walk forward you can force him to go with you, and you have so much leverage upon him that he cannot swing around and use his left hand in defence. This trick should prove of value in ridding one's home or office of an annoying caller with whom it is not necessary to use very much ceremony. He will go, depend upon it, if urged in this fashion.

There are almost endless methods of applying this trick of "bending the arm the wrong way." By exercising his ingenuity the student will be able to devise many combinations, several of which will be found to impress any man whose sense of humour in not impaired by the fact that the joke is on himself.

CHAPTER XIII

A CLEVER JAPANESE WAY OF EXPOSING
S H A M M E D UNCONSCIOUSNESS — THE
SHOULDER PINCH AS A MEANS OF DE-
FENCE—A HANDY WAY OF STOPPING A
FIGHT IN A SECOND—AN ATTACK FROM
BEHIND THAT LEAVES THE VICTIM WITH-
OUT DEFENCE, AND ITS APPLICATION TO
A BURGLAR OR OTHER INTRUDER

IN a system of combat where strategy is as
highly developed as it is in *jiu-jitsu* it is to
be expected that the student will have to deal
with the problem of shamming by his opponent.
Indeed, the *jiu-jitsian* never hesitates to sham
when by so doing he can gain any advantage.

The only shamming that is regarded as being
dishonourable is for one contestant to pretend
to surrender, and then to take instant advantage of the cessation of his punishment by
making an unlooked-for attack upon his adversary. But shammed unconsciousness is a trick

in which no surrender has been proclaimed. If the victor in a bout can be deceived into believing that his victim has been rendered unconscious, and if the victor is lured thus into relaxing his vigilance, it is wholly proper to take advantage of his carelessness.

For this reason it often becomes necessary to know whether an opponent is only pretending to have been deprived of his senses. The method of investigating that is shown in photograph No. 26 is an ingenious and effective one, and has the further excuse that it will restore consciousness in light attacks of fainting as well as in severe "attacks" of feinting.

The assailant throws himself on the ground beside his adversary. With the tips of one finger the aggressor jabs the suspected pretender lightly and repeatedly in the solar plexus, while the investigator's other hand is employed in giving the shoulder pinch. The unremitting jabs in the plexus are in themselves enough to fill a shammer with a very lively desire to leap to his feet and thus deliver himself from the nauseating, nerve-wracking prodding. And the pain caused by the shoulder pinch completes the pretender's earnest desire to escape further torment by surrender.

It takes but very little time for the student to make himself master of this shoulder pinch. The thumb is pressed into the front side of the top of the shoulder, while the grip is kept by grasping with the fingers at the back of the shoulder. A very little practice upon his own shoulder will show a *jiu-jitsian* just where the spot is that is hyper-sensitive to the pinch with the thumb. Bear in mind that the ball of the thumb should dig in at the point where the head of the upper arm joins the scapula.

Having learned this shoulder pinch, it be-hooves the student to experiment for the purpose of learning in how many combinations it can be used with effect. It is useful often in a clinch at close quarters, causing the adversary to wriggle out or to draw away from a punish-ment so painful. While the pinch leaves some soreness in its wake the feat is by no means a disabling one, and it may be resorted to as often as it is needed in attack or defence.

Often this pinch can be employed by itself and not in combination. If the assailant secures a good grip in this fashion, keeping his own body as far away from return attack as possible, the victim is often forced to draw back out of striking distance.

In photograph No. 27 a possible complication is shown. Here one of the contestants has bent swiftly forward to the ground in order to strike a sharp edge-of-the-hand blow against his opponent's shin. The latter, divining the intention, has promptly resorted to a shoulder pinch that will destroy the effect of the hand blow. For a little experimenting with severe shoulder pinches will show that this form of attack deprives an opponent's arm of nearly all of its striking power.

Still another value of this shoulder pinch will be suggested to the investigating student. Often, in a throw, the victim will fall upon one side. It is an advantage to the aggressor to have his man lying face downward. In that case the shoulder pinch should be applied roughly to the shoulder on the ground. The pain is so intense that the victim rolls over on his face in order to weaken the force of the pinch. If he does the assailant must take prompt advantage by kneeling with one knee in the back of his opponent and the other knee across the back of one of the upper arms of the prostrate one.

Now, the wrist of the arm that is so pinned must be seized, and the arm forced upward with a strong pull. As the upper portion of the arm is pinned by a knee, and the front side of the arm is downward, the victim's arm is forced through that painful process of which so much has been said, the process of "bending the wrong way." And the result of this ex-cruciating torment is unconditional and prompt surrender on the part of the now helpless victim.

Still another way of taking this shoulder pinch is for the assailant to approach from be-hind and to seize both his opponent's shoul-ders, this time placing the thumbs at the backs of the shoulders and digging with the fingers into the sensitive spot at the front of the shoulder. It is a torturing form of punish-ment that prompts the victim, instinctively, to kick backward with his heels, and the aggressor must be on the alert to prevent damage to his own shins. If this backward kick with the heel is attempted the aggressor must promptly accomplish either a trip or a knee jab in one of the victim's kidneys.

Again, when this spot on the front of the shoulder has been located so that the *jiu-jitsu* student can strike it unerringly, it is to be borne in mind that it offers an excellent point of attack for an edge-of-the-hand blow. The effect of this blow is to lame the arm so much that the victim's desire to continue the contest in greatly lessened.

If ever troubled, in a crowd or in a narrow passage-way, by an obstinate fellow who can, but who will not, give you an opportunity to go forward, try the effect of the shoulder pinch from behind on both shoulders, at the same time pushing him ahead of you. He will go in the desired direction. And the same applies to any one who is to be ejected from the premises.

With a good-natured friend the shoulder pinch, lightly applied from behind on one shoulder, is an amusing way of forcing him to turn and face you. In actual combat, of

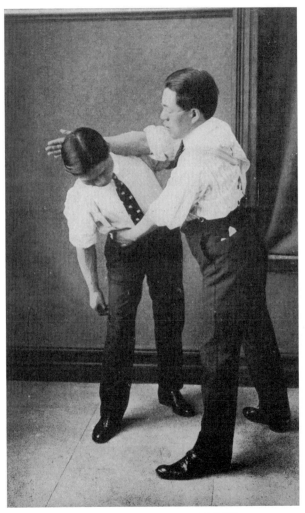

No. 30. AN UGLY BACK-OF-THE-NECK BLOW.

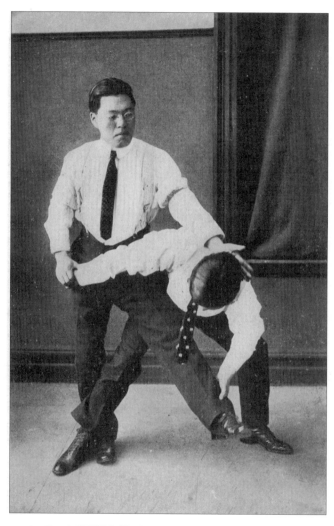

No. 31. A POSSIBLE COMPLICATION IN SIMULTANEOUS ATTACK.

course, it is never an advantage to make an opponent face you, as the attack, if it can be begun from behind, is much better finished in that position.

In the feat illustrated by photograph No. 28 we come to a trick that may be played upon an opponent from a position at his side. This is another application of "bending the arm the wrong way." Seize his nearer wrist with both hands. At the same time thrust your nearer foot in front of his nearer foot, hooking it. His wrist must be held with the inside forward. When seizing the wrist a pressure downward on his arm forces him to bend forward. Pull the arm across your nearer leg, and with the pressure at his captured wrist bend the arm backward. If it is wished the attack can be ended in a throw, tripping his engaged foot and completing the work with a wrench on his captured arm. If the victim be taken properly he cannot offer any saving counter, and, even without the throw, he is reduced to prompt surrender.

This same principle may be applied in a slightly different fashion. Seize his wrist as before, but do not attempt to make the victim bend forward. Instead, raise your nearer knee, planting it firmly against the back of his upper arm. And the hold is much more firmly taken if one hand only is employed in seizing the enemy's wrist, the other hand gripping at his shoulder. Some of the effect of the shoulder pinch may be had in gripping the shoulder.

All thought of further fight will leave the victim who is severely attacked after the method that is illustrated by photograph No. 29. This trick may be practised safely enough between friends, employing light blows, but it is hardly to be recommended in actual combat save where the circumstances justify ugly attack.

Both arms of the aggressor are used simultaneously, but in order to enable the student to get at the idea piece-meal the work of the arms will be described separately. One hand is jabbed fairly over the kidney, in the soft part just below the last rib. This attack on the kidney is delivered with great severity when actual combat calls for it. The jab may be delivered with the finger tips, or with the clenched fist. Or it may be given very effectively with the middle knuckle of the second finger projecting from the clenched fist. It is highly important that the blow be struck just at the most sensitive point. The effect is to make the victim feel "sick all over." It "takes ambition out" of him. In any style of attack a severe kidney blow has the same effect, utterly weakening the man who receives it.

The fore-arm of the other arm is struck back smartly upon the jugular. Some practice must be undertaken in order to make this blow effective to its utmost. If the "Adam's apple" be struck, instead of the jugular, the effect is that much the more disastrous to the victim, but it is easier to land with full force on the jugular.

The effect of this attack is, of course, to throw the victim backward. Thus, at the moment of the double striking, the assailant should spring backward and allow his man to strike the ground. The victim will be so weak that the assailant will not be called upon to use the utmost nimbleness in following up the attack by reducing his opponent to complete submission.

The illustration shows with exactness the relative positions of the two contestants.

CHAPTER XIV

TWO EXCELLENT COMBINATION ATTACKS FOR
EXTREME OCCASIONS—HOW TO STOP A
PASSING FUGITIVE IN THE STREET—HOW
TO OVERTAKE A FUGITIVE AND REDUCE
HIM TO SUBMISSION

SEVERAL hints have been given already as
to certain edge-of-the-hand blows that,
while they should be given lightly in friendly
bouts of practice, should never be employed
in actual combat except under stress of dire
necessity. In other words, these dangerous
blows should not be resorted to in any condition of encounter where the *jiu-jitsian* would
not feel equally justified in using a deadly
weapon.

These dangerous blows are those that may
be struck against the "Adam's apple," slantingly across the temples, horizontally just over
the ear, and at the base of the brain. The
blow on the "Adam's apple" is not deadly.

125

but he who uses it runs the risk of smashing the hyoid bone, and thus of doing irreparable injury to the vocal apparatus and to the swallowing processes. As has been explained before, the blow over the jugular will answer every purpose of defence as well. Blows on the temples, or just over an ear are likely to result in serious and lasting brain injury. Even an edge-of-the-hand blow at the base of the spine, if delivered with too great force, is likely to cripple the recipient for life.

But the most dangerous of all these blows is that at the base of the skull. It may cause death. The concussion of the blow may result in injury to the medulla oblongata of so serious a nature as to stop the action of the heart and lungs, and thus put an end to life itself.

None of these dangerous blows would have been mentioned by the author but for the fact that the student, in experimenting, would be very likely to find them out for himself and to employ them in ignorance of the consequences. With this premise we will pass to the consideration of two tricks that may be employed in cases of extreme personal danger. Photograph

No. 30 illustrates the first of them. Here the
assailant employs his left hand in taking a
momentary body-hold at his opponent's right
side. This blow may be taken squarely at the
side, but should be in the soft part below the
last rib, and should be delivered with as much
force as the assailant can employ for the impact. The aim in striking hard at this point
is to incapacitate the victim as much as possible
at the outset. If the relative positions of the
two combatants permit it is even better that
the blow be landed over the right kidney, but
this would require a rather wide reach around
the victim's body when the second half of the
attack is made.

Instantly after striking at the right side the
assailant should employ his own right hand in
delivering a sharp edge blow at the base of his
adversary's skull. If both hands of the aggressor are used with sufficient smartness and
force the collapse of the victim is instantane-
ous. Skill in this feat should be acquired by
all women students as it will be of value to
them in any case where they are attacked in
the absence of their natural protectors. And

a woman is peculiarly able to use strategy in the use of such a trick. A male assailant would not look for effective resistance from a woman, and in the first few seconds of surprise she can pretend shrinking fear, throwing the would-be assailant off his guard. Then like a flash she can dispose of the intruder. If she plants her blows skilfully and forcibly there will be no immediate need of a police officer's presence. There will be time enough for her to get her breath and to take a parting look in the glass before setting out in quest of a blue-coat.

As much may be said for the situation that is suggested by photograph No. 31. Here the assailant begins the attack from the opponent's side. The first move is to seize the victim's nearer wrist with the hand of the arm that is farther from the victim. This wrist is to be held in a tight grip until the victim is prostrate. The victim shown in the illustration, at the moment that his wrist was seized, has bent swiftly forward to seize his opponent's leg, near the ankle, for the purpose of making a throw. This, however, renders it all the easier for the aggressor to follow the capture

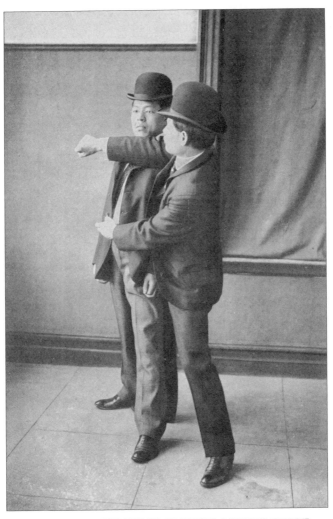

No. 32. ONE JIU-JITSU METHOD OF HALTING A RUNNING FUGITIVE.

of the wrist swiftly with a blow at the base of the skull—and the encounter is ended!

Once or twice in a lifetime it may happen that a citizen will have occasion to stop a fugitive fleeing through the streets. The same need may arise with a policeman several times in a month. It is an easy matter to stop a fugitive from behind, for, in running he is at his worst for self-defence.

Of course, if he is running away from you, the first matter is to catch up with him. Unfortunately in this detail *jiu-jitsu* has no help to offer. All depends upon the pursuer's sprinting abilities, and the running track is the best place to acquire speed.

But, if you can overtake your fugitive, the simplest plan is to throw both arms around his neck, clasping one wrist with the other hand at the front of his throat. Stop the instant that you have the hold. In the next second spring back, dragging the fellow to the ground.

There is another way of doing the thing, which consists in seizing the fugitive by the shoulders. Throw your right leg in front of his right leg, and throw him over your leg.

In chasing a fugitive it must be always borne in mind that merely seizing him is not a safe programme. The throw must follow instantly. Even though he seems a man of slight physique, the fugitive may be master of some dangerous fighting tricks. If he is merely caught and held he is likely to make use of some trick whose least effect will be to leave the pursuer behind, hopelessly humiliated over a defeat for which he had not looked.

There is another way in which a fugitive can be stopped from behind, and it is so effective that it is worth a good deal of practice. The chances are that the pursuer will be wearing either a coat or a jacket. As he sprints after the fleeing fellow let him strip off this garment, holding it in readiness in both hands.

At the instant of overtaking the fugitive throw the garment over his head, enveloping it, and make the garment fast by gripping it tightly in a hold around his neck. Then, as the victim is dragged back to the ground, his head is closely enveloped. Unable to see anything, his chances of fighting effectively are reduced to next to nothing.

In case the fugitive halts and turns quickly, try to throw the garment over his face before he can prevent the attack. In this position, too, his inability to see what his assailant is doing to him will make defence much more difficult.

How shall a fugitive be stopped by a citizen toward whom he is running? Ninety-nine men out of one hundred would, under these circumstances, make the effort by thrusting a foot sideways and tripping the fellow. But this method has its dangers. The writer remembers a case that occurred in San Francisco more than a dozen years ago. A Chinaman, after having committed a murder in the street, took to his heels with a howling mob pursuing. The murderer was fleet, and seemed to have a fair chance of getting away.

Up the street, in the opposite direction to that taken by the fugitive, came a young Italian. He saw the Chinaman coming toward him, pistol in hand, and with the mob behind. Taking in the situation, the Italian halted for an instant, then, as the Mongol went by, thrust out a foot to trip. Quick as a flash the Chinaman raised his weapon and fired. The bullet went into the Italian's leg. Swerving but a foot or two, the Chinaman kept on without having abated his speed for an instant. Had it not been that a young man fleet of foot joined the mob behind and set a swift pace, the yellow criminal would have gotten away for the time being.

Of all ways for stopping a fugitive who is running toward you is that which is depicted in photograph No. 32. As soon as you catch sight of the runner make up your mind just what is to be done and do it coolly. The situation calls for strategy. Continue your pace toward the fugitive, neither slackening nor increasing your speed. Do not seem to be looking at him at all.

If you act the part well the fugitive will not plan any attack upon you. He has just gotten himself into trouble, and he does not want any more. He sees nothing suspicious in your conduct and keeps on. The whole thing happens in a few seconds.

Just as the fugitive is passing—when it is too late for him to act against you—throw out your nearer arm, catching him across the abdomen. Hold on tightly. In the same instant swing around so that your farther arm may be employed in striking him squarely across the front of the throat.

The hold at the abdomen has checked the speed of the runner, and, of itself, will almost stop him. But the blow across the throat sends him backward at the very instant when his speed has been greatly lessened. The result of this double attack is that the fugitive goes over backward. The *jiu-jitsian* who has read this far in the book with profit will know just how to secure his man when he has sent him to the ground.

The very act of stopping the runner when going at full speed has all but destroyed his balance. It requires but a little more of impulse to carry him wholly off his feet. Fall upon him, securing, if feasible, a hold that will enable you to make his arm "bend the wrong way"—and the fugitive will find his career stopped as thoroughly as if he had collided with a stone wall.

CHAPTER XV

THE student who has mastered all of the work that has been described in the foregoing chapters will have a good basic knowledge of the most important principles of *jiu-jitsu.* What more he has to learn will come mainly from practice and from a trained observation that will enable him to make the utmost use of what he has learned.

One can rehearse the tricks given in this book, and he will have a good theoretical knowledge of the ancient Japanese art of protecting himself. But the practical knowledge is needed in its highest degree, and this can come only from keeping up the work, and from learning to use each trick with an agility that is ever increasing.

At the base of all true *jiu-jitsu* are good nature and leniency. The adept in *jiu-jitsu* must never be a bully; he must not go about with the proverbial chip on his shoulder. He must not seek trouble, but should do all that he sensibly can to avoid encounters that are anything more than friendly. Cultivate patience and good nature. If a dispute threatens to lead to personal encounter do not make the first move of attack until it becomes unavoidable.

A Japanese who is versed in the snares of *jiu-jitsu* is better equipped for fighting than any man can be who is not so equipped. Yet the Japanese are proverbially polite and they are patient to an extreme. The Japanese who is threatened by a bully does not immediately set himself in aggressive action. Instead, he smiles, and does his best to smooth the difficulty over. Back of his smile lurks the consciousness that no man but a *jiu-jitsian* of greater skill than his own can by any possibility defeat him. When one knows in advance that he is to win in an encounter he can afford to be patient.

It is time, now, for the student to practise
with some one who is familiar with Anglo-
Saxon methods of attack.   The student should
learn all of the ways in which he is likely to be
attacked.   The most popular form of attack
with an Anglo-Saxon is to let his fist fly
straight out from the shoulder.   This the
student knows how to stop by catching the fist
and "breaking" the assailant's arm over his
own shoulder.   Probably this is the most important single feat for use in encountering a
boxer.   The student must take pains to get well
past the theoretical stage in this performance.
He should render himself, through constant
practice, letter-perfect in the use of the trick.
Never be satisfied with the speed that has been
gained; always strive for better and better
speed.   It is well, though, to bear in mind that
it is a cardinal rule in boxing that a counter
can be employed, if it be a good one, in slightly
less time than is required for the assault.

But, in practising this trick of catching the
opponent's fist, do not overlook the importance
of the fendings that may be made with the
edge of the hand against an assailant's arm.

Do not neglect practice in this style of defence, which is of great value in stopping a blow when there is not time to get the hands up for catching a fist.   The edge-of-the-hand blows are useful also in a variety of cases where the contestants are at close bodily quarters.

Then, when the opponent ducks as he strikes, one must always be prepared to catch the head in the *jiu-jitsu* of chancery that has been explained.   This chancery is highly effective, and is far safer than the back-of-the-neck blow that would naturally suggest itself to the novice in *jiu-jitsu*.   And with the enemy's head in chancery the hand not employed otherwise can be made to do a finishing piece of work in the form of a kidney blow.

A method of attacking a man that is employed much in this country consists of rushing at him, securing him by both shoulders, or by the upper arms, giving him the back heel of wrestling, and throwing him to the ground. This can be met promptly, and stopped effectively by the *jiu-jitsian ;* for the latter has one of his hands at the assailant's back.   Here there are two ways in which the *jiu-jitsian* can defend himself. One is to employ his elbow in a jab at the short ribs of his assailant. Usually this blow can be delivered with great severity, and it can be landed at the instant that the aggressor has taken hold. The other method is for the *jiu-jitsian* to use the hand that is at his enemy's back in a kidney blow. Very often an alert man on the defensive can use both blows at the very instant that the aggressor takes the clinch. In that case it is certain that the assailant will not make a throw. It is a favourite trick with some rough and ready fighters to rush forward, duck and seize the intended victim with one arm thrust under the crotch, then rising with the victim and throwing him. Sometimes this can be met by the agile *jiu-jitsian* with the Japanese form of chancery hold. It can always be countered, if the man on the defensive is as agile as he should be, by dropping both hands on the back of the aggressor's head as he ducks, thus making it impossible for him to rise. And one hand can be swiftly released by the man on the defensive and applied to the assailant's kidney on the nearer side.

It is well, too, for the *jiu-jitsian* to remember
that he should never be satisfied with one defensive blow when two or three can be used in
rapid succession. Study out how many blows
may be used in swift sequence and with disconcerting effect on the antagonist. Suppose,
for example, that the two antagonists are in a
clinch with their nearer sides close together.
The *jiu-jitsian* is able to inflict an elbow jab in
the enemy's short ribs; this may be followed,
like a flash with three other moves—a finger-
tip jab in the solar plexus, an edge-of-the-hand
blow under the point of the chin, and a slanting
edge-of-the-hand blow on the forehead. The
enemy who receives all of these styles of attack
in the space of some three seconds will not feel
like fighting any more that day. It is well
worth the student's while to practise this sequence, and to devise as many more as he can
by intelligent practice of what he has learned
in other feats. In especial the student should
remember to follow the solar-plexus jab always,
when practicable, with an edge-of-the-hand
blow under the point of the chin. In this case
it is always the thumb side of the hand that

is used, the thumb being folded across the palm.

In rough-and-tumble clinches it is a favourite trick to use the knee against the crotch or the abdomen, and if the *jiu-jitsian* permits himself to be caught unawares in this fashion he is all but sure to be defeated. When a clinch is to be made, always swing one side of the body toward the assailant, keeping the nearer leg in such position that the aggressor cannot land with his knee either in the crotch or in the abdomen. This knack can be acquired with a little practice. This position has the added advantage of enabling the *jiu-jitsian* to use his own knee where his enemy has not taken a similar precaution.

In some parts of Europe it is a favourite trick, in beginning an impromptu fight, for the aggressor to lift one arm in a defensive position and to try to drive the steel ferrule of his umbrella or cane into his antagonist's abdomen. This nasty trick is not by any means unknown in this country. Yet the defence against this form of attack is an easy one, calling mainly for well-developed agility. Take a side step

swiftly to that side of the opponent's body
that is farther from the cane or umbrella.   At
the instant of taking the step land an edge-of-
the-hand blow on the enemy's jugular, en-
deavouring to make this blow forcible enough
and sharp enough to send him to the ground.
At the instant of landing, or trying to land,
the blow take a second side step.   The idea of
this second step is that, in case the blow fails
to land properly, you have carried yourself out
of reach of your opponent.

Then there is the assailant who comes up
behind and who wraps his arms around his
intended victim, pinning them at the latter's
sides.   In one of the earlier chapters of this
volume the student has been told how to free
himself from this hold, following it with an
elbow jab in the abdomen.   But it is possible,
also, to throw the assailant, if he seizes you in
this fashion.   First of all, free yourself parti-
ally from his hold, after the manner advised
when the elbow jab is used.   Follow the free-
ing by seizing one of his legs and straightening
up, just as the policeman has been advised
to do when employing the counter to the

club trick. And, in general, the policeman's method of ridding himself of his tormentor is applicable in every case of being seized from behind, except in the case of the hold that is illustrated in photograph No. 22. Where the *jiu-jitsian* is himself the assailant from behind he is advised to employ this latter form of hold in every instance where it can be used.

When attacked with a straight-out kick, of course the method of defence should be to catch the coming foot just back of the heel, jerk the foot upward, and send the aggressor over on his back. But this style of kick is so easily met and countered that it is seldom attempted in real combat.

It will repay the student well who has gone thus far to study out all possible forms of attack that are outside of *jiu-jitsu*, and to study next what the most effective kind of *jiu-jitsu* counter would be. With the groundwork of Japanese tricks that has been given the student who does the most thinking and practising will be the most formidable opponent, for the student has reached a point now where he can and should become his own instructor—ever watchful and alert in practice, and ever remembering that through practice the performance of every feat should be as second nature.

CHAPTER XVI

FINISHING TOUCHES IN THE JAPANESE SCI-
ENCE OF ATTACK AND DEFENCE—A SUM-
MARY OF THE BEST FEATS FOR WOMEN
TO PRACTISE AND TO USE AT NEED—
FINAL CAUTIONS TO THE STUDENT WHO
WOULD BE EXPERT IN "JIU-JITSU"

I T is in acquiring the finishing touches of the
ancient art that the student shows whether
or not he is naturally fitted for expert work in
jiu-jitsu. Every feat that he performs is based
on some natural law, and the extension and
perfection of the feat depend upon the students' ability to observe natural laws and to
apply them.

For example, when striking downward with
an edge-of-the-hand blow the student should
discover that the blow is both more easy and
more effective if the weight of his body be
added to the impulse. Then a little thought
will show the *jiu-jitsian* that by springing

slightly off his feet just before landing with his hand the weight of his body will be added to the blow.

After a very little practice the student will find that this knowledge and its application has greatly increased his efficiency. It will then occur to the student that a brisk forward impulse will add to the value of any blow or jab he may use in frontal attack. He must study, now, how to give that forward impulse.

In the same manner he will find out for himself just how to make his weight count for the most when trying to bear down an opponent; and he will learn how to straighten up with the weight of the opponent on his back.

No indications for the solution of these problems are to be offered to the student now. If he cannot solve them for himself, after a little effort, he may know that he is lacking the instincts that make the true *jiu-jitsian*.

Not very many years ago it would have been considered, in this country, an impertinent thing to suggest that women should learn these combat tricks, or at least the simplest and most serviceable of them. But of late years the athletic woman has begun to develop a healthful interest in the lighter work of boxing and wrestling, and so it is natural that she should continue her education in the matter of physical encounter, and become something of an expert in *jiu-jitsu*. It was in London that women first fell in with this idea, and Japanese instructors became suddenly in great demand. The craze quickly crossed the ocean, and in the United States, to-day, there are not a few women who are capable of holding their own in combat with men.

Several of the feats that the author has described in the present volume may be learned readily by women, and should be used by them at any time of need and in the absence of their natural protectors. The edge-of-the-hand blow over the jugular is one that is easy of acquirement by women. The hold that is secured by bending the arm up behind the back is another feat that should be practised by women. The "come along," and, in fact, many of the applications of "bending the arm the wrong way" are of especial value to women who do not think it beneath their dignity to be able to defend themselves at a pinch.   And every woman who feels the slightest interest in the subject should persuade herself to practise repeatedly at the trick of stopping and catching an assailant's fist and of "breaking" the attacking arm over her shoulder.

And especially effective for women are the jabs that may be delivered with either elbow in the short ribs of an opponent, or in the soft parts just below.   If a woman is annoyed by a fellow who steps up to her side in a crowded street it does not come amiss to know how to give him an effective elbow jab in the solar plexus or in the abdomen.   The woman who can do this neatly will save herself from further annoyance.

Any of the holds or throws that have been explained in these pages will be of service to the woman who finds an intruder in her home at a time when its natural male protectors are away.   But, as the average American woman of athletic tendencies is still a trifle backward in the desire to learn throws she will content herself at present with mastering a few holds, and be satisfied with this method of securing an intruder. Here is a simple hold that will serve for the detention of a thief or insolent rascal until her cries bring a policeman or a neighbour:

For the purpose of practice, stand at the left side of the practice opponent, and a little to the rear at the same time. The intended victim should stand with his arms hanging naturally at his side. The student thrusts her left arm between his left arm and the body, and at a point barely above his elbow. Her left arm is forced horizontally across his back.

Now, at the same instant, her right hand pounces upon his right elbow, and that arm is forced over towards his left. Her left hand seizes his right arm just above the elbow, while her left elbow hooks with his left elbow. The hand that is resting forcibly on his right elbow forces this right arm over to where it can be seized.

It is easy, then, for the woman assailant to hold the victim's arms behind his back with her left arm and hand, and her right hand still on his right elbow keeps his right arm in place. In addition, she is able to release her right

hand for the striking of a blow if it becomes
necessary.

With some practice any woman of ordinary
strength can acquire the knack of seizing and
holding a man in this fashion. She can take
him quite unawares and render him helpless
without the outlay of much exertion. She
must, however, look out that he does not succeed in kicking back with his heel, and, if he
does try it, she must be prepared to strike or
to choke with her right hand, which may be
spared for the purpose.

There are many other feats in *jiu-jitsu* that a
woman may learn to employ with most convincing embarrassment to a male assailant, and
the author would suggest that all the tricks of
combat that he has described be experimented
with by our American women and by their
English sisters, and that the most attractive be
thoroughly mastered. If a feat in combat is
needed by a woman but once in her lifetime,
yet is ready when the moment comes, it is
worth all the cost of effort in learning it.

A few words of final caution, if they are heed-
ed, will be of value to the student of either sex.

In the first place, do not be eager to learn too much at the outset. One feat, *mastered*, is worth a half-dozen that are but half-learned. It is far better, in the beginning, to take up but one trick, and to keep at that until the performance of it is natural and easy for the student. Then devote the same amount of effort to a second trick. When the two are well mastered, practise them alternately during a few bouts, then adding a third, and, after a few days more, a fourth trick. This may seem tedious to the student, but it will repay him well where he will meet only with ultimate disappointment if he gives way to the rather natural impulse to pick up at least a dozen feats during the first bout of practice.

Patience, steadiness, thoroughness pay heavy dividends in the study of *jiu-jitsu*. Four years is the average length of time devoted to the study of the art in a Japanese school.

Care must be taken not to carry the effort to the wearying point in any one practice bout. The body may not suffer, but *jiu-jitsu*, in its best development, is subtle and crafty, and the active mind can be tired very easily. When the fatigue point for the brain is reached, all further practice in that bout is detrimental to the student's practice. Twenty minutes in a day is enough time to devote to practice, if the student's mind be kept keenly on the alert. The practice bout should never last longer than a half an hour.

If it can be borne in mind, at all times, that the bout should be even more of a mental than a physical drill, then the best results will be obtained. In *jiu-jitsu* extreme discipline of the mind is both a requirement and a result.

THE END